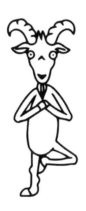

GOAT YOGA

THE LIGHT IN ME
HONORS THE GOAT IN YOU

SHENANIGOATS YOGA AND ASHLEY HYLBERT

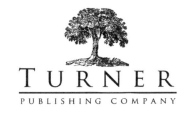

TURNER
PUBLISHING COMPANY

Turner Publishing Company
Nashville, Tennessee
New York, New York
www.turnerpublishing.com

Goat Yoga: The Light in Me Honors the Goat in You

Book design: Maddie Cothren
Photography: Ashley Hylbert
Illustrations: Brandon Henderson

Library of Congress Cataloging-in-Publication Data available from the Library of Congress

Printed in the United States of America
17 18 19 20 10 9 8 7 6 5 4 3 2 1

CONTENTS

MEET THE AUTHORS

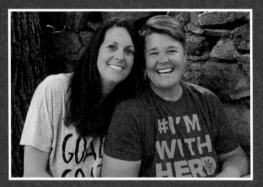

SHENANIGOATS YOGA

is based in Nashville, Tennessee and began in June of 2017. The owners, Jamie Codispoti and Max Knudsen, have a gorgeous indoor studio that hosts goat yoga classes, bachelorette parties and private events. The Shenanigoats team travels throughout middle Tennessee allowing those outside of Music City to experience their magic. Shenanigoats Yoga was recently rated the number one thing to do while in Nashville by the *Tennessean*. Their goats have kicked off PR summits for hotels, mingled with Grammy award winning singers, reality TV super stars, bridesmaids and birthday girls... and to them, a flat back to jump on is all that matters. Jamie and Max feel strongly about making every class one that is filled with laughter and fun; they focus on customer service and will never tire of hearing, "This is the best day ever!"

ASHLEY HYLBERT

is a Nashville-based photographer and exercise addict with a sweet tooth. She grew up in Aspen, Colorado and received a degree in communications from Ithaca College. Earlier in her career she worked in publishing for Conde Nast in San Francisco and *Tatler Magazine* in London.

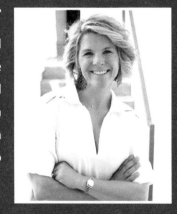

For Kendall and JD, may kindness and laughter always guide your path.

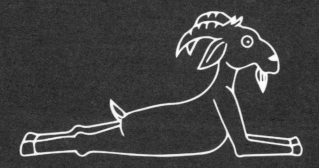

To my fun, free-spirited daughter—Annie Hylbert.

INTRODUCTION

A QUICK NOTE FROM SHENANIGOATS YOGA:

Why Goat Yoga?

The word yoga means "union," so why not unite with our four-legged friends? Aside from being a lighthearted and unique experience, the health benefits of interacting with animals are well documented: it decreases cortisol (the stress hormone) levels, while increasing oxytocin (the feel-good hormone) and dopamine, a neurotransmitter. With that trifecta of internal chemistry, plus the added bonus of genuine laughter, people can't help but love the experience and cherish the memories.

With millions of people practicing yoga worldwide, the variations of its practice and study are always expanding. Some yogis who come to our classes are traditional in their practice and seldom deviate from their routine, while others are open to anything that brings peace and a sense of well-being to their mat—even if it's a baby goat hopping joyfully around them! People do yoga for many reasons; for some it's the physical challenge, for others it's to escape—just for an hour—the city and noise around them; or perhaps it's the tool they are using to heal. Yogis show up to class after a hectic day, and many times say, "I wasn't going to come because my day was so crazy, but I had to see the goats."

Goat Yoga is not your typical practice. It's about connecting with animals, finding balance amid distraction, focused and intentional movement, spending time with friends, and laughter. So. Much. Laughter!

 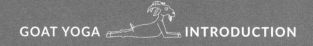

RUMINATIONS ON GOAT YOGA

Do I have to be experienced at yoga to do Goat Yoga?

Not at all! Some of the goats are beginners as well. Goat Yoga is about laughter, light exercise, and experiencing animals and yoga in a new way. You do not need to be experienced in the poses to reap the benefits of this class.

So, is it a "real" yoga class?

Participants are encouraged to interact with the goats before and after class, but it is impossible to complete a class without giggles and "selfies." Attendees should expect to have fun connecting with the goats and experiencing poses in a new way—often with a goat atop them! There are many wonderful flows that are enriched with the addition of goats as you will see in this book, and even the most experienced yogis will be challenged to hold poses longer because of sleeping goats or photo ops!

What should I bring to Goat Yoga?

You should bring a mat that you do not cherish, a towel, bug spray, bottled water, a cellphone or camera, and you should leave your ego(at) behind. Contrary to popular belief, goats cannot eat everything, so treats should be provided to class participants by those who know the goats best.

What should I wear to Goat Yoga?

When it comes to skin, less is more! Goat hooves can be scratchy, so make sure to not leave sensitive skin exposed. You will likely find yourself trying new poses and will constantly be taking photos, so make sure to wear comfortable and stretchy exercise clothing. Leave your expensive yoga clothes at home, and since some goats enjoy snacking on jewelry, it's best to avoid accessorizing.

Do yoga goats bite?

A good "rule of thumb" is keep your fingers to yourself. While goats are friendly animals, they are mischievous and always on the hunt for a good nibble, but yoga goats are certainly not aggressive. Baby goats, especially those that have been bottle fed, will often try to nurse fingers and toes.

Do all goats have horns?

Most goats are born with horns. Many farms practice disbudding, where the horns are removed while the goat is young. They do this for a variety of reasons, mostly for safety and so goats don't get caught in fences.

Will they pee or poop on my mat / me?

In short—possibly. While you should try to be vigilant and quick on your feet, accidents do happen and sometimes they happen on people. Goat Yoga should always be practiced with ready access to vinegar, towels, and bleach wipes for those occasional mat spills. Healthy goat poop comes in tiny pellets like rabbit or deer poop and it's very good for your lawn, so if your class is outside just sweep it aside.

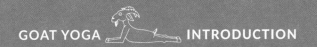

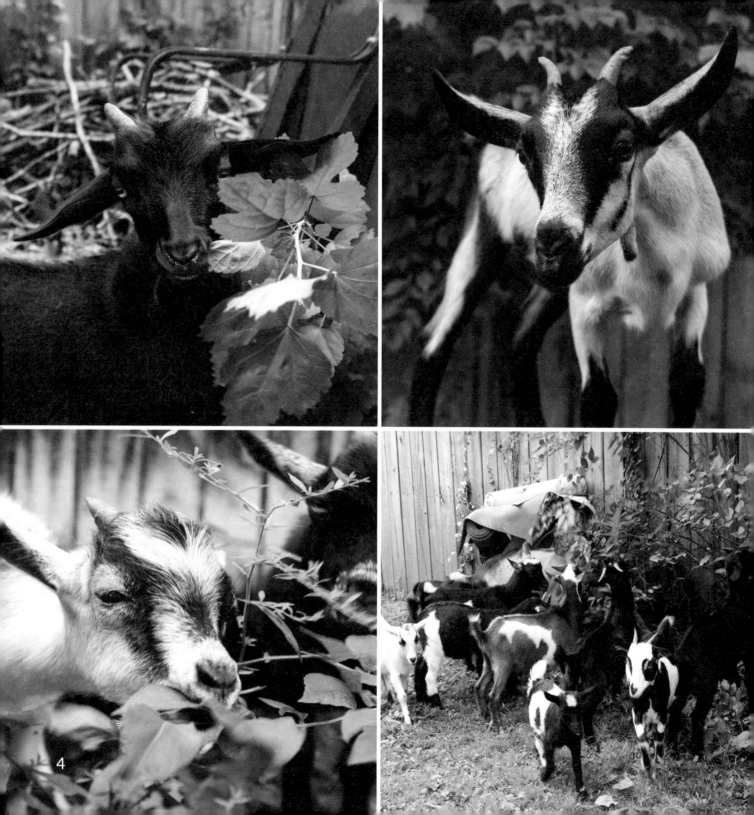

4

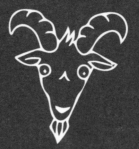

ROUNDING UP THE HERD

Goat and Yogi Bios

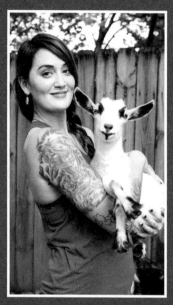

GILLIAN

Gillian began her asana practice in 1999 and went on to open Steadfast and True Yoga in Nashville, TN in 2010 with the goal to create a studio and space that holds tightly to values of right action and less distraction to create healthy reactions.

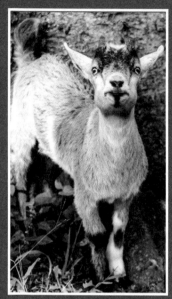

MILES

Age:
3 months
Breed:
Nigerian Dwarf
Known for his piercing blue eyes and his love of heights, Miles is a fan favorite and has his own Instagram account!

Follow him @IAmMilesTheGoat

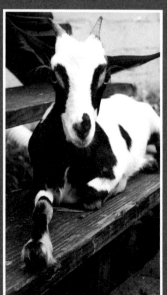

SHEEP

Age:
8 months
Breed:
Nigerian Dwarf/ Myotonic hybrid
This tri-colored beauty got her name because her mama's name is Bo Peep.

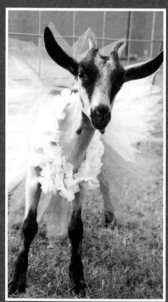

PENELOPE

Age:
6 months
Breed:
French Alpine
Favorite Pose:
the goat circle

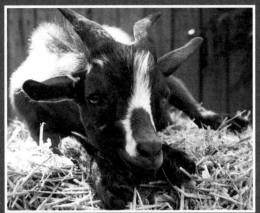

NOAH

Age: 6 months
Breed: Nigerian Dwarf/Pygmy hybrid
Noah was brought to life by the farmer who gave him mouth-to-nose resuscitation after his birth!
Noah shamelessly stole the earring of an unsuspecting yogi! Only one stolen earring to hundreds of stolen hearts.

LORI

Lori made the transition from student to teacher in early 2012 and practices BarreAmpled, Bounce and Yoga. When not teaching, she can usually be found outdoors with her husband and dogs—most likely barefoot.

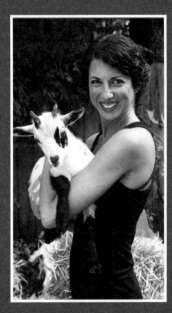

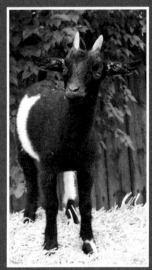

MAC

Age: 6 months
Breed: Nigerian Dwarf
Mac loves any yoga pose that he can leap off of! He's known for his fancy, gold-medal worthy dismounts.

MUSH

Age: 4 months
Breed: Pygmy
Mush came to Shenanigoats from Alabama and was very timid, but now he loves to be held and his yoga skills are really amping up!

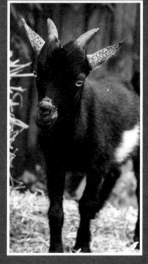

BALLER

Age: 3 months / Breed: Pygmy
Baller has been a wild man since birth. He loves spending time with his mama and jumping on tables any chance he gets!

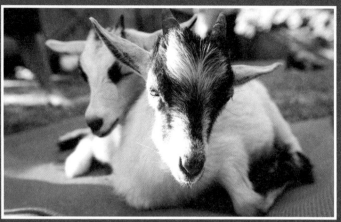

BELLA & CHARLIE (TWINS)

Age: 5 months
Breed: Nigerian Dwarf/Pygmy hybrid
Charlie always looks like he's got some extra food stuffed away in his cheek and has earned the nickname of 'Chubby Cheeks Charlie.' The pair can often be found cuddling together.

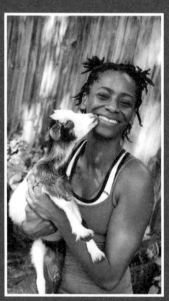

RENEE

In 2014, Renee created RW Yoga in the hopes to get people, especially women of color, to understand that there is more to yoga than the physical aspect. She encourages them to understand the discipline, openness, love and internal growth that goes along with yoga.

ROOTBEER FLOAT

Age: 3 months
Breed: Pygmy
Rootbeer loves to cuddle and is known for her big belly, teeny stick legs, and crooked tail.

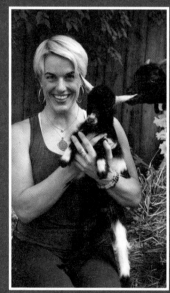

SARA JANE

A decade long yoga practitioner and a yoga teacher for the last 5 years, Sara Jane didn't know she loved acro until she tried it for the first time three years ago. She is a skilled flyer and a strong base who always wants to practice a skill just one more time.

LIBERTY

Age: 3 months
Breed: Pygmy
Liberty was born on the 4th of July!

WILL

Born in Grand Rapids, MI, Will attended Columbia College for Music and Theatre before developing a passion for yoga. One of his favorite mantras is: "You have to find your edge in order to push it further."

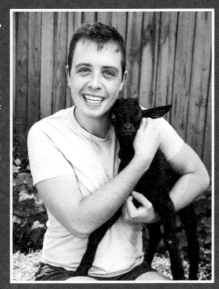

FRANK SINATRA

Age: 5 months
Breed: Nigerian Dwarf
Frank got his name for those Sinatra eyes. He enjoys rocking a great outfit.

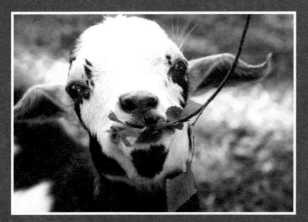

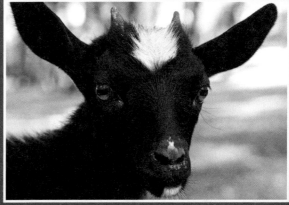

HARVEY MILK

Age: 5 months
Breed: Myotonic (Tennessee Fainting)
Harvey is named for one of our real-life heroes! He's less rambunctious than the others and loves to pick a special yogi and share their mat for the duration of class.

ROBBIE WASABI

Age: 3 months
Breed: Pygmy
Robbie loves car rides and snuggling. She has the perfect square patch of white hair on her forehead.

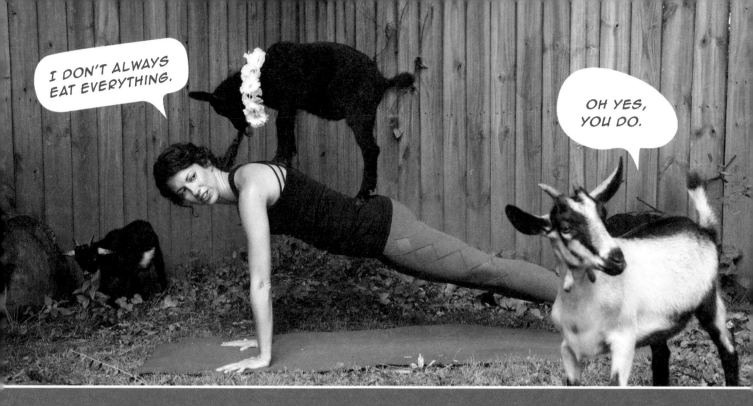

A NOTE ON THE GOATS:

Goats (caprine) are the epitome of agility and balance. If you have never seen a goat jump up a steep cliff or balance on seemingly impossible terrain, we encourage you to do so. They are herd animals and do best when they interact with other goats.

Our goats are the most important element of our practice. Their care and handling is fundamental to enjoying a holistic, healthy, and safe experience. Most goats enjoy the challenges presented by the shapes of yoga and will enthusiastically leap from yogi to yogi, but if one becomes tired or disinterested in being part of our yoga classes, it is retired to our landscaping crew. If you are interested in goat yoga, look locally for family farms that value the care of their animals.

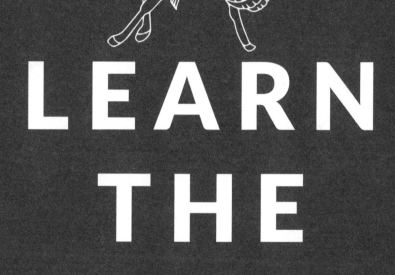

LEARN
THE
FLOW

Poses and Flows with Goats

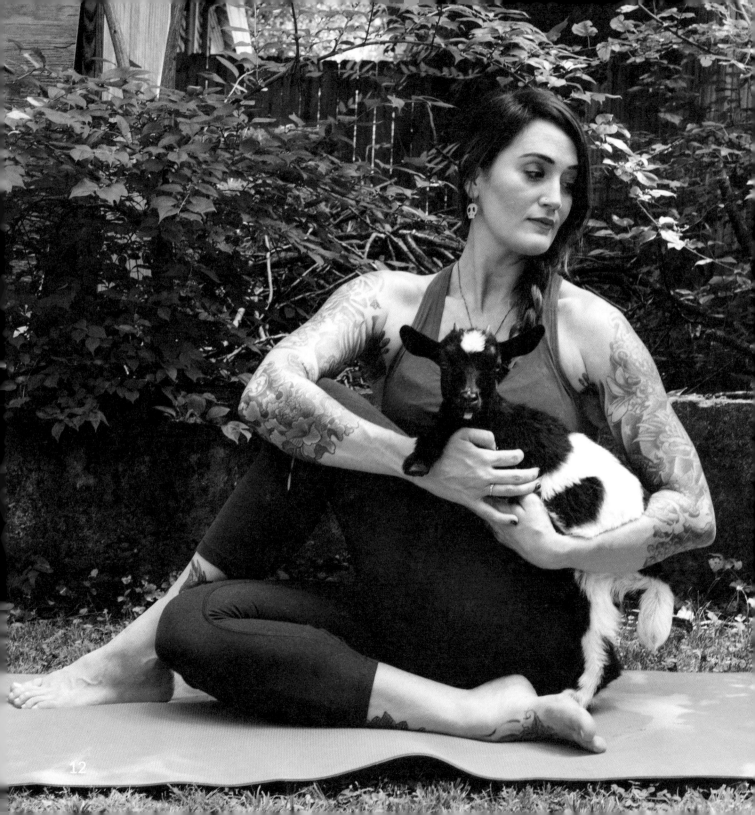

HALF LORD OF THE GOAT

(Half Lord of the Fishes)

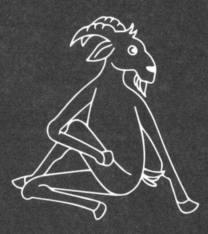

A great twist and perfect pose for goat cuddling!

Seated on your mat, bend one knee over the other, hugging the top knee close to your chest. Then reach for the nearest baby goat and hug him too.

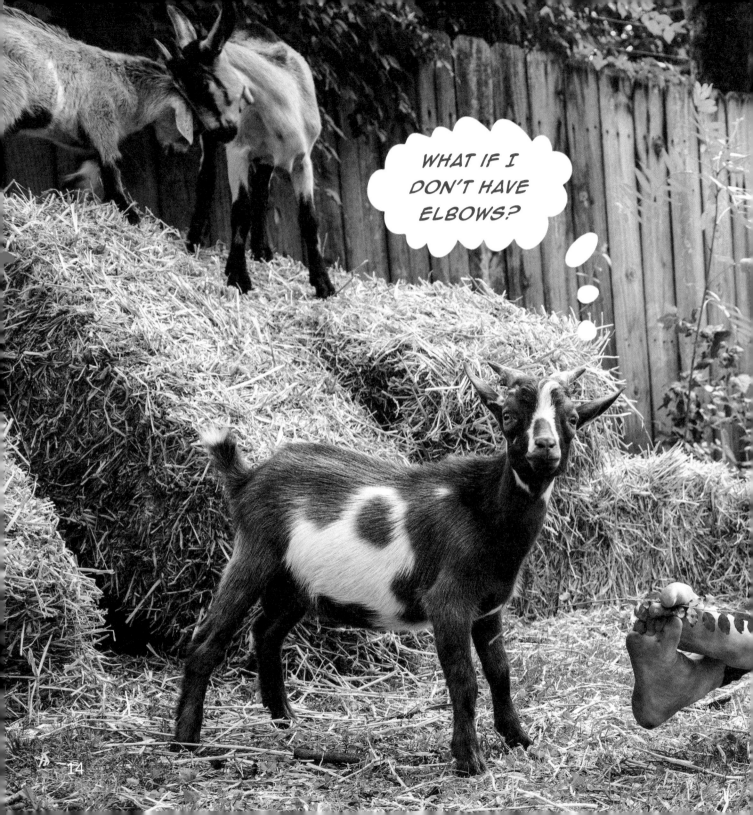

FLYING GOAT
(Eight Angle Pose)

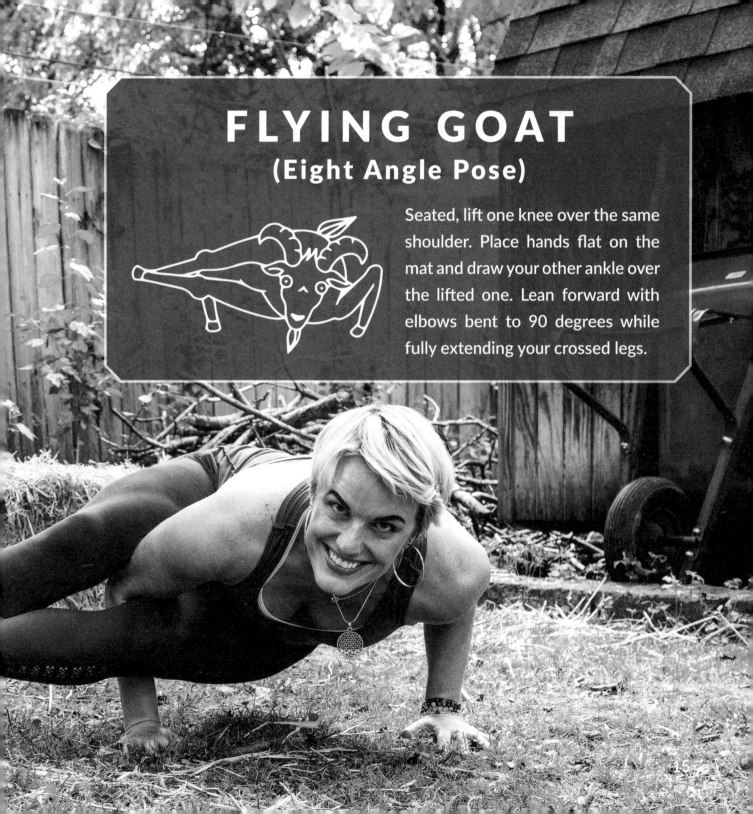

Seated, lift one knee over the same shoulder. Place hands flat on the mat and draw your other ankle over the lifted one. Lean forward with elbows bent to 90 degrees while fully extending your crossed legs.

RAM-EL

(Camel)

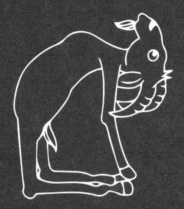

A great pose when you need to have a good heart-to-hoof with a friend. Start kneeling with toes tucked and heels lifted. Lean back, reaching your hands to your ankles. Press the hips forward and reach chest high, lastly allow your head to fall back to a comfortable place. Option to untuck the toes for a deeper backbend. (Recommended for less hefty goats and less busty yogis.)

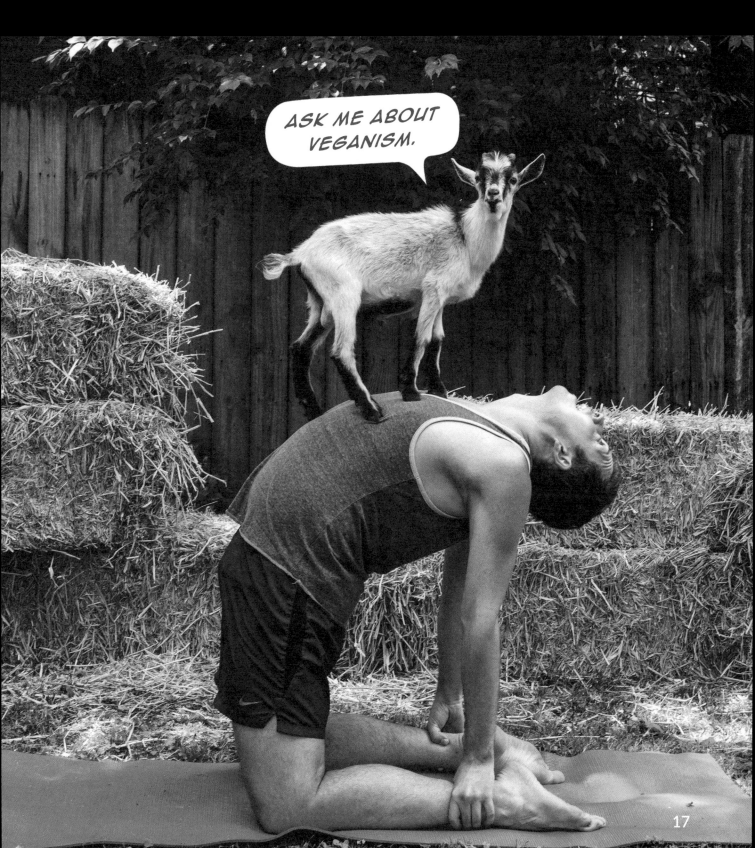

17

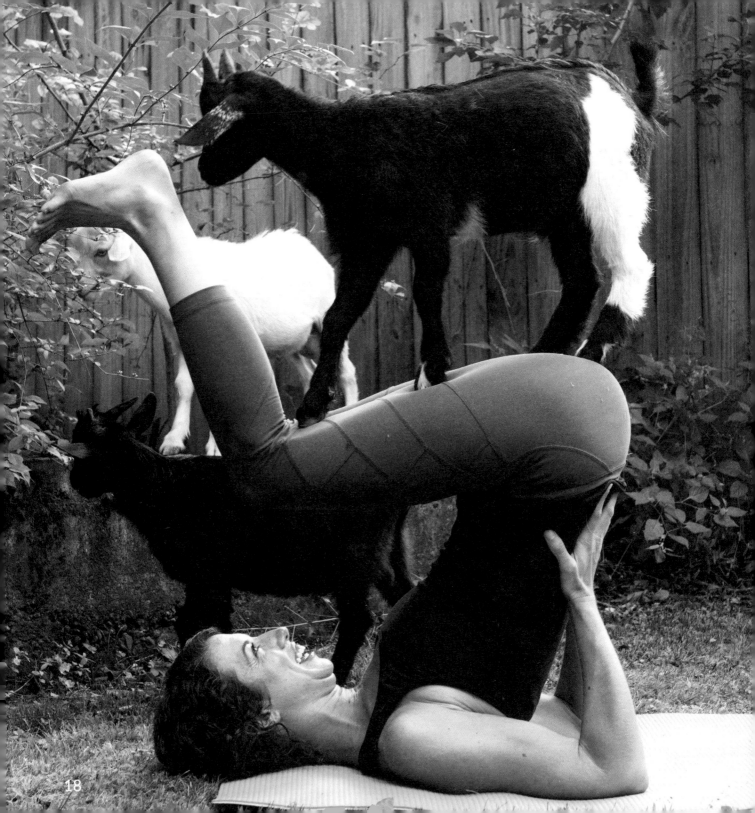

GOAT STAND

(Shoulder Stand)

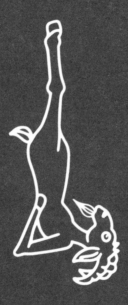

A variation on shoulder stand where your legs are bent to protect your face from sharp goat toes. Lying on your back, draw your knees into your chest, and bend your legs to lift them over your head. Hands are used to support the lower back. Make sure you avoid putting weight on your neck.

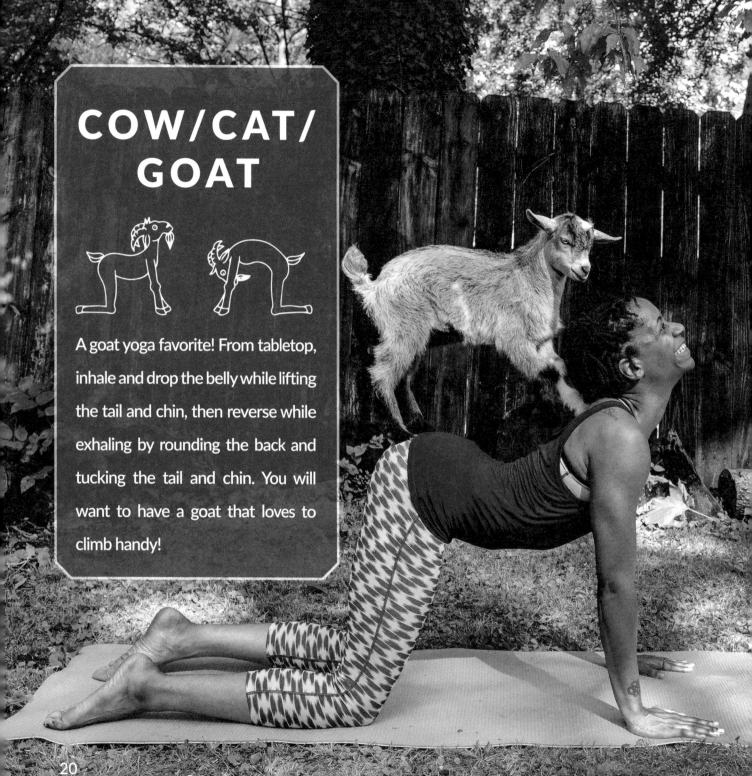

COW/CAT/ GOAT

A goat yoga favorite! From tabletop, inhale and drop the belly while lifting the tail and chin, then reverse while exhaling by rounding the back and tucking the tail and chin. You will want to have a goat that loves to climb handy!

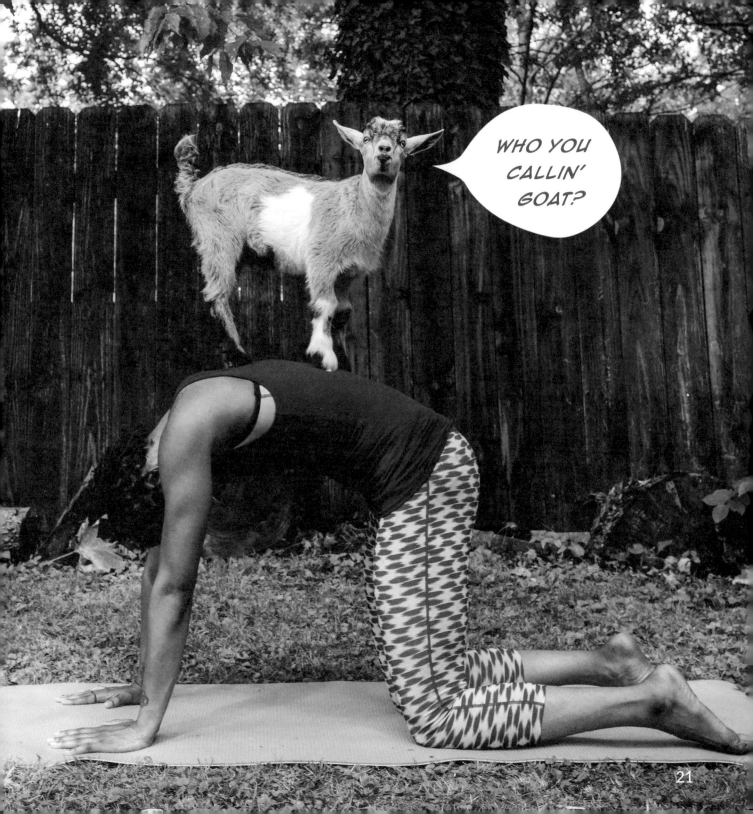

21

BOTTLE KONASANA
(Baddha Konasana)

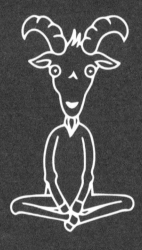

A thoroughly restorative pose when you have a bottle baby goat handy! Sit with the soles of the feet together and knees out wide with a bottle in one hand and a thirsty goat in the other!

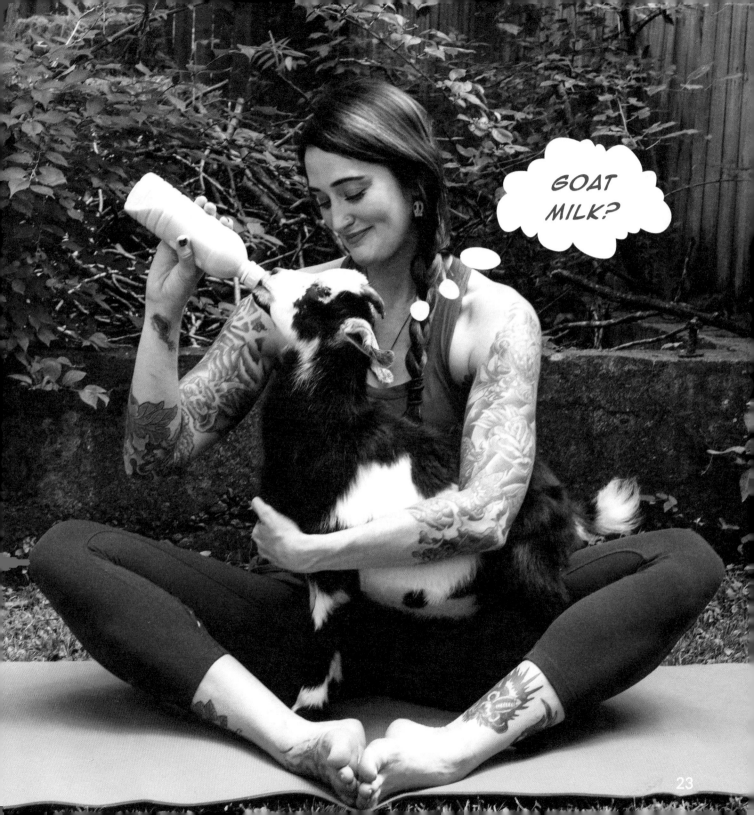

DOWNWARD FACING GOAT

(Downward Facing Dog)

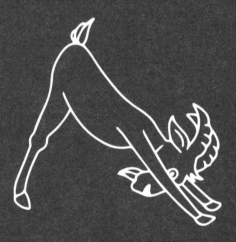

Most Goat Yoga classes will have at least one goat that favors this pose—and it is great for photo ops! From tabletop position, tuck your toes and press your arms straight, lifting your hips up while letting your head relax between your arms.

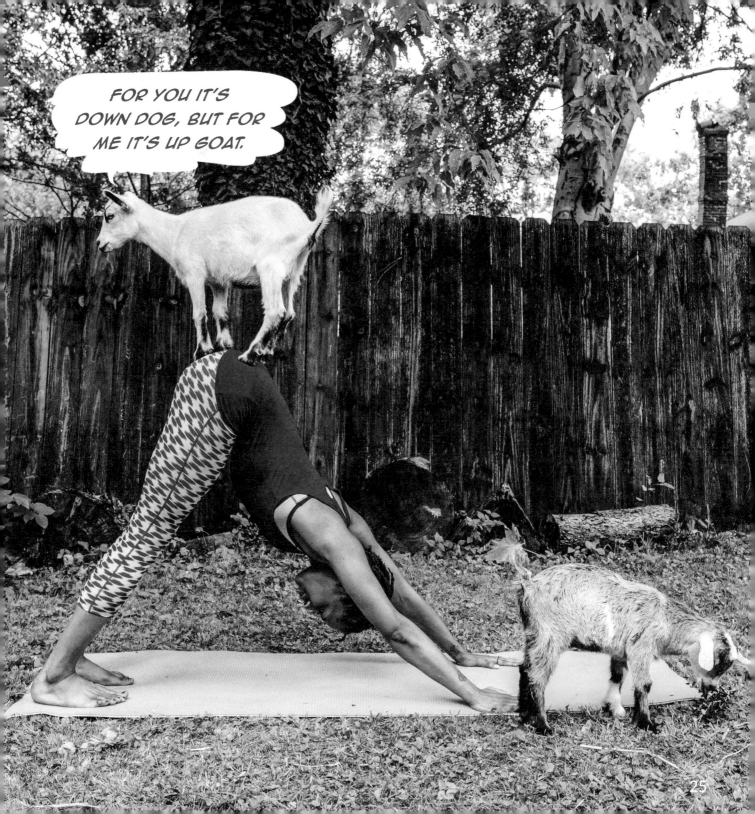

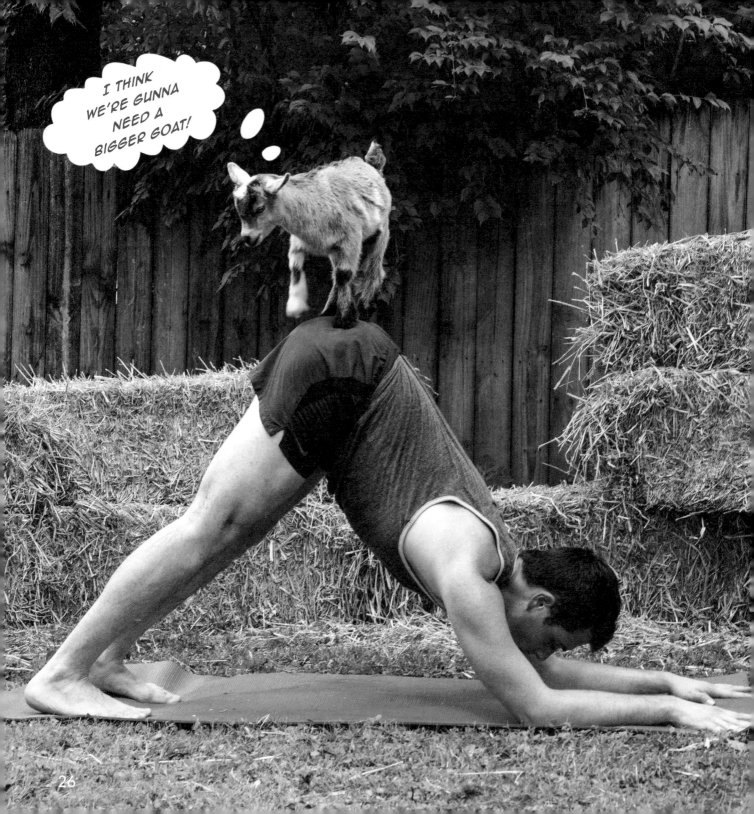

GOAT OF THE SEA

(Dolphin)

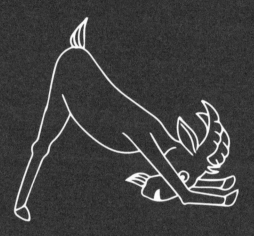

An advanced variation of Downward Facing Goat (page 24).
While keeping your balancing goat in place, drop your elbows
to the ground and keep them parallel while letting your head
rest to the ground or look forward.

UPWARD FACING GOAT
(Upward Facing Dog)

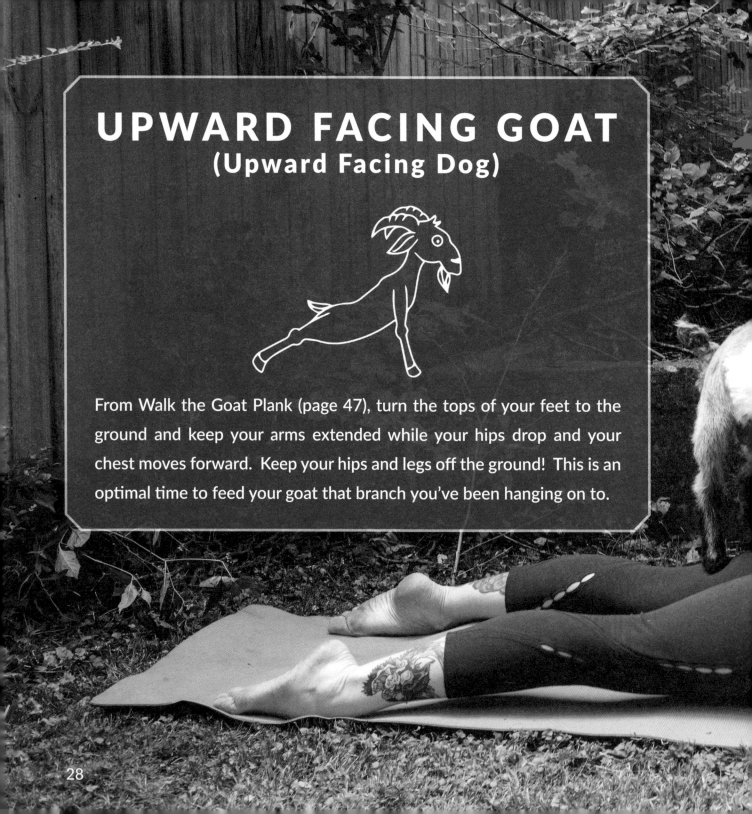

From Walk the Goat Plank (page 47), turn the tops of your feet to the ground and keep your arms extended while your hips drop and your chest moves forward. Keep your hips and legs off the ground! This is an optimal time to feed your goat that branch you've been hanging on to.

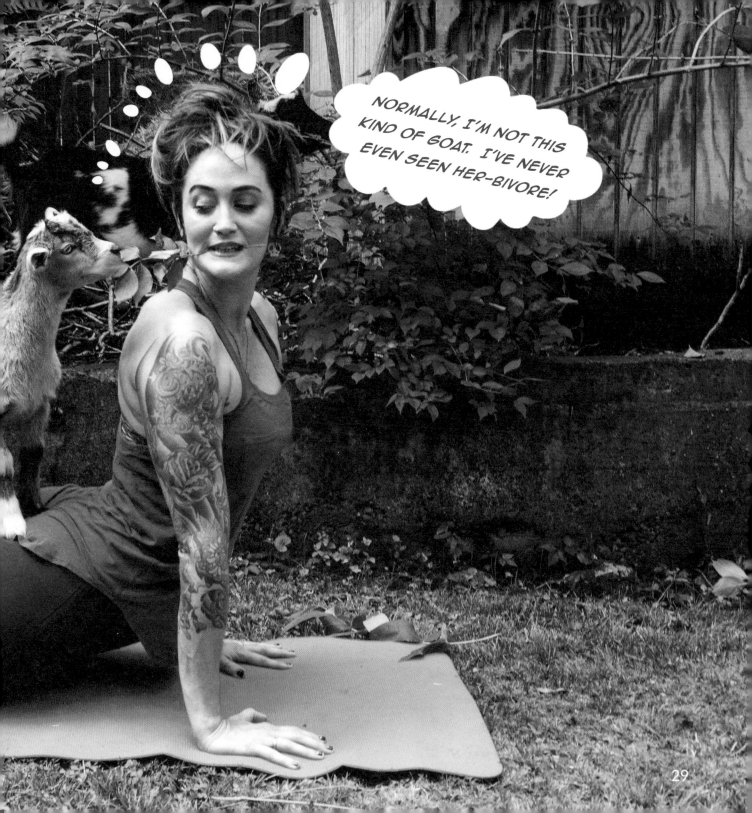

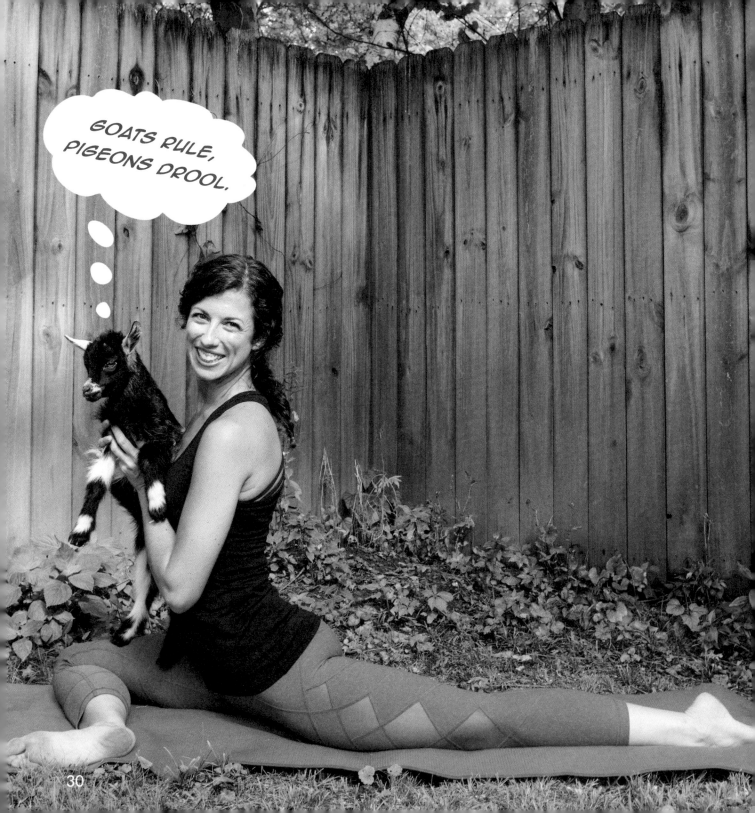

EKA PADA
GOAT-ASANA

(Pigeon)

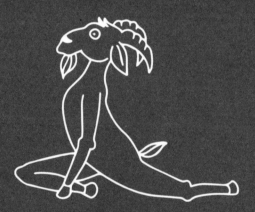

A great stretch for your hips and haunches. For the upward variation, goat hugging is encouraged, while bending forward over your bent leg will inevitably lead to happy goat climbing—just watch your hair!

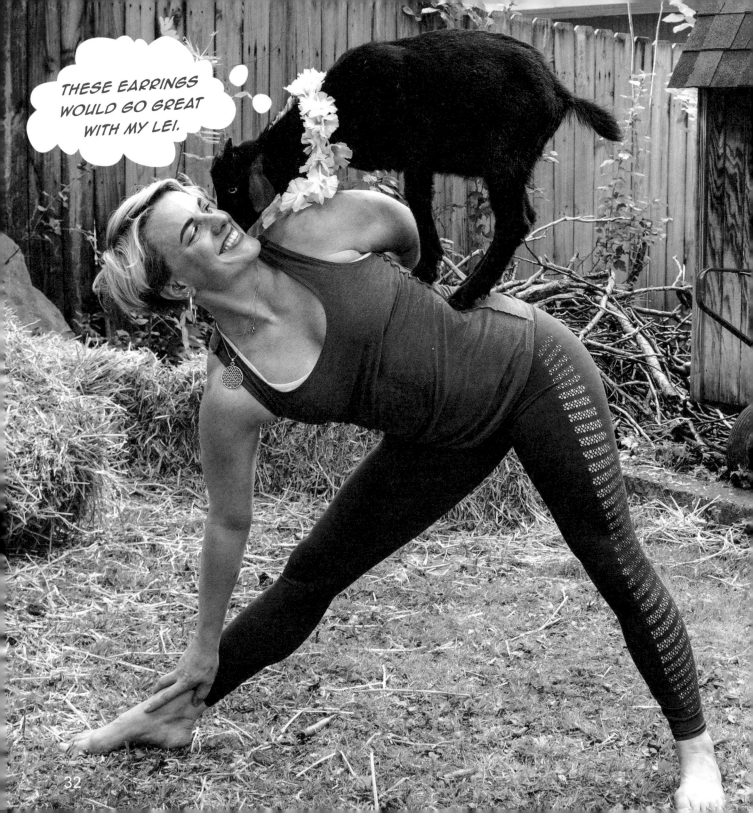

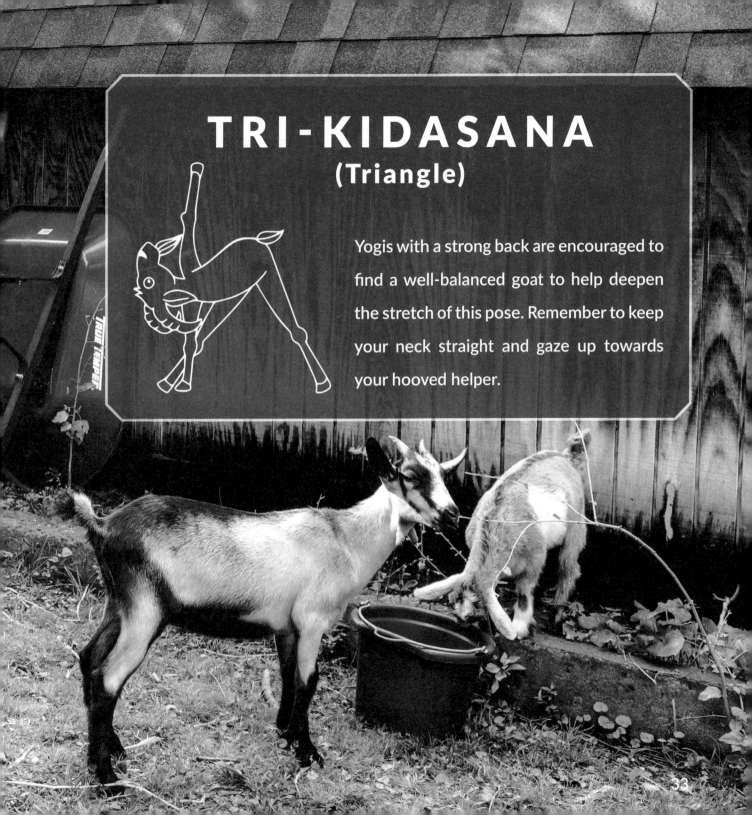

TRI-KIDASANA
(Triangle)

Yogis with a strong back are encouraged to find a well-balanced goat to help deepen the stretch of this pose. Remember to keep your neck straight and gaze up towards your hooved helper.

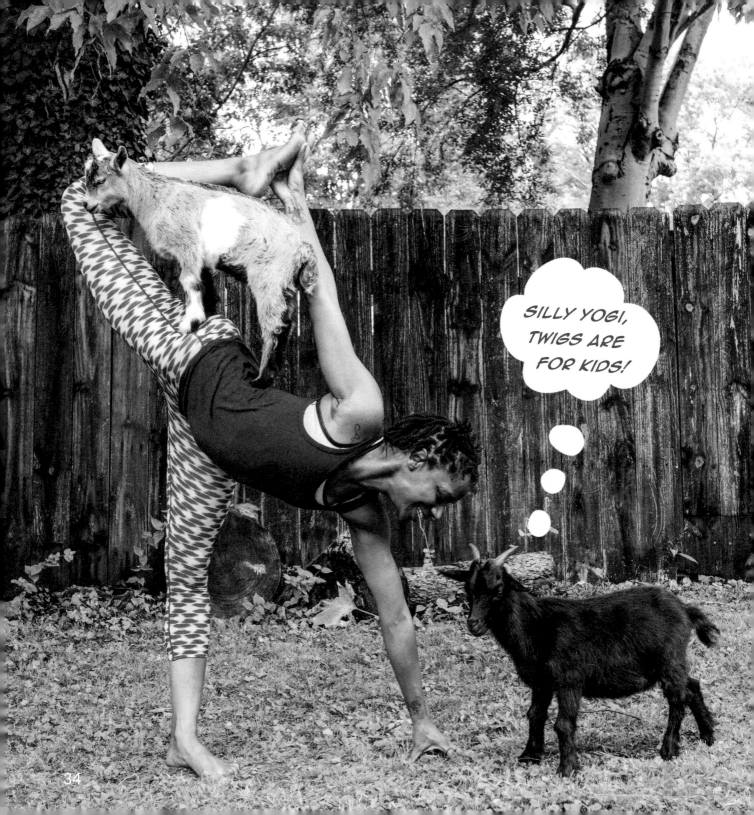

MOON GOAT

(Half Moon)

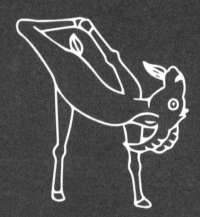

This footbound variation of half moon gives the goat more support and the yogi a better counter balance to help hold that goat up high! From standing, bend forward with one hand reaching to the ground while the opposite leg reaches towards the sky. Remember to keep a flat back and look forward for balance.

HAY WHEEL

(Wheel)

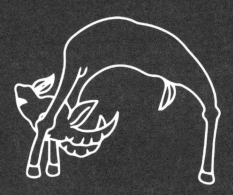

This energizing pose is another great way to show off your best goat. From lying on your back, place your palms down by your ears and press the floor to lift your torso until fully extended. To come out of this pose, tuck your chin and lower down to your back—but make sure to check for goats below!

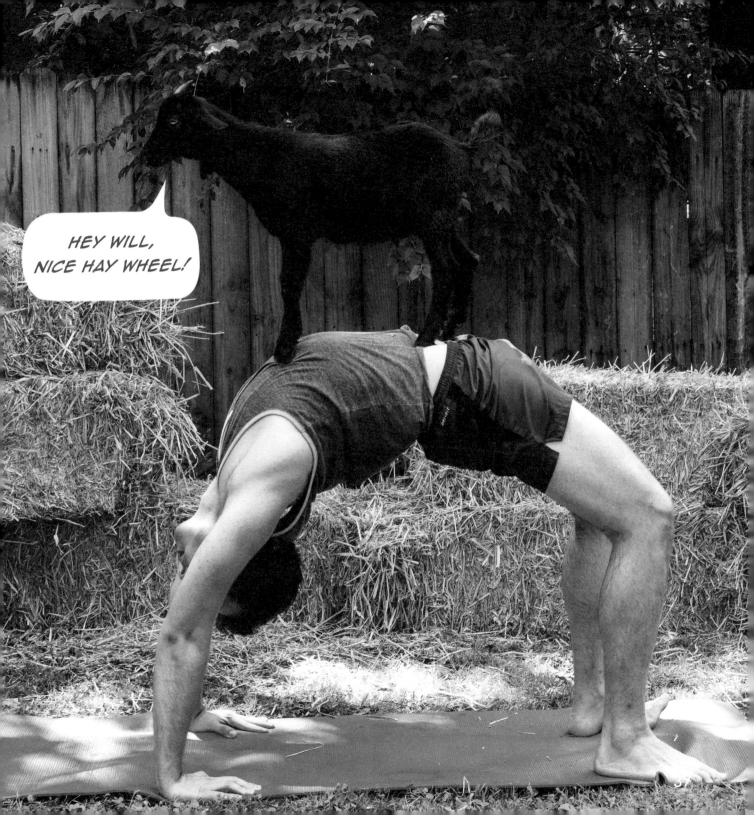

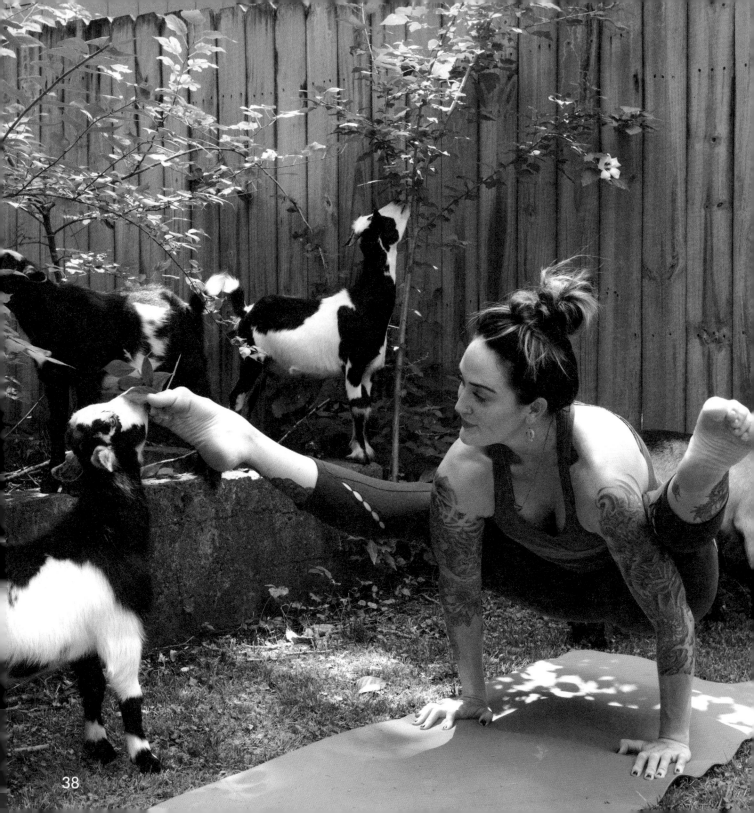

TITIBAAAAASANA

(Firefly)

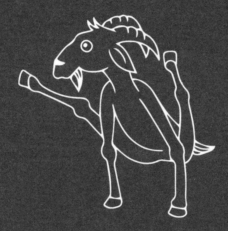

This balancing pose requires more core than arm strength and should be practiced around hungry goats that won't shy away from eating twigs from your toes. When lifting, reach through the point of your toes to straighten your legs—which is actually made easier by gripping a leafy treat for your cloven friend.

WALK LIKE AN EGYPTIAN

(Sphinx)

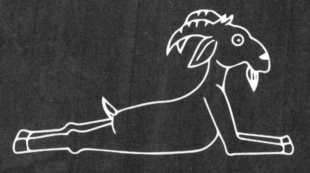

Resting on your forearms and releasing your lower back, you will find it easy to crack a smile as you come face-to-face with the kids.

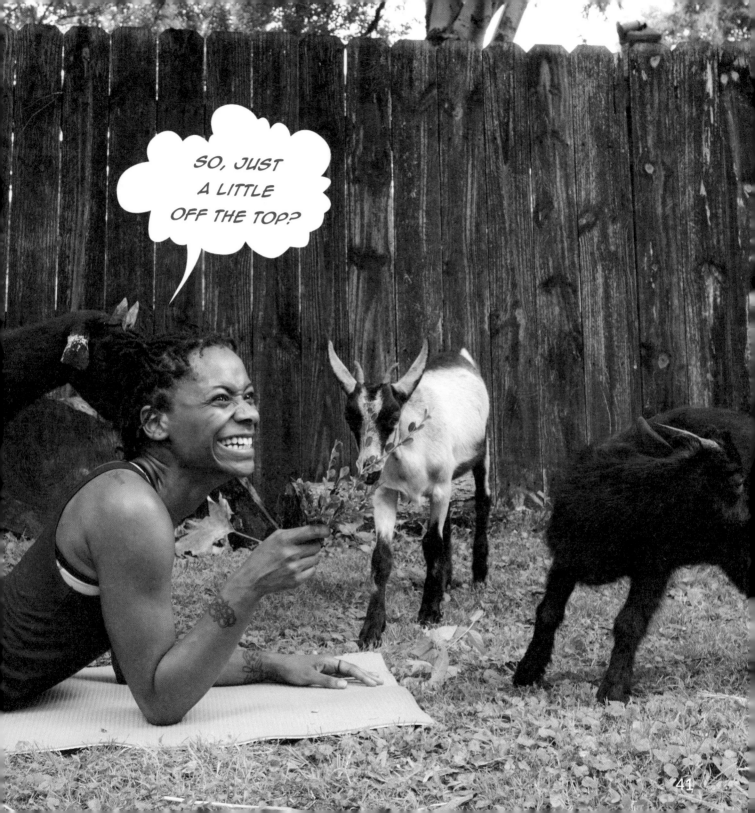

DANCING WITH GOATS

(Dancer)

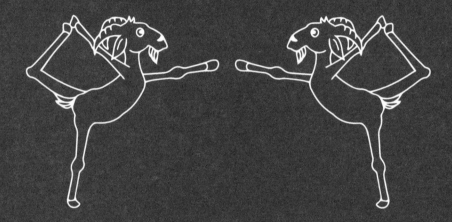

Goats love a good hug! The stretch and depth of this pose are increased by the counterbalance created by goat cuddles. With a strong standing leg and a goat in one arm, extend your free arm behind you to grab the corresponding leg and bend forward only when your foot reaches the height of your shoulder. Just be aware—you will never out-dance a goat.

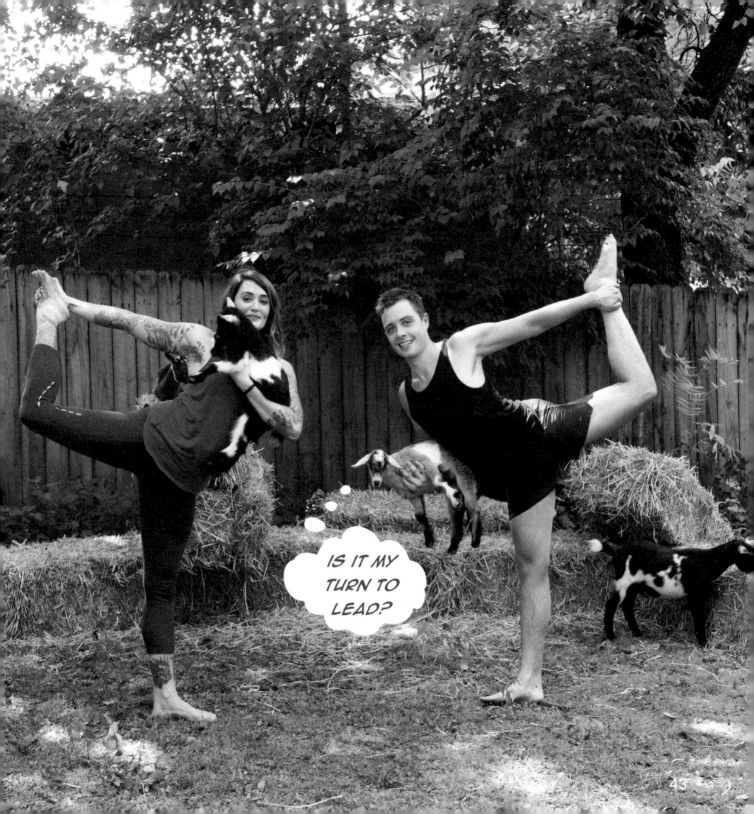

43

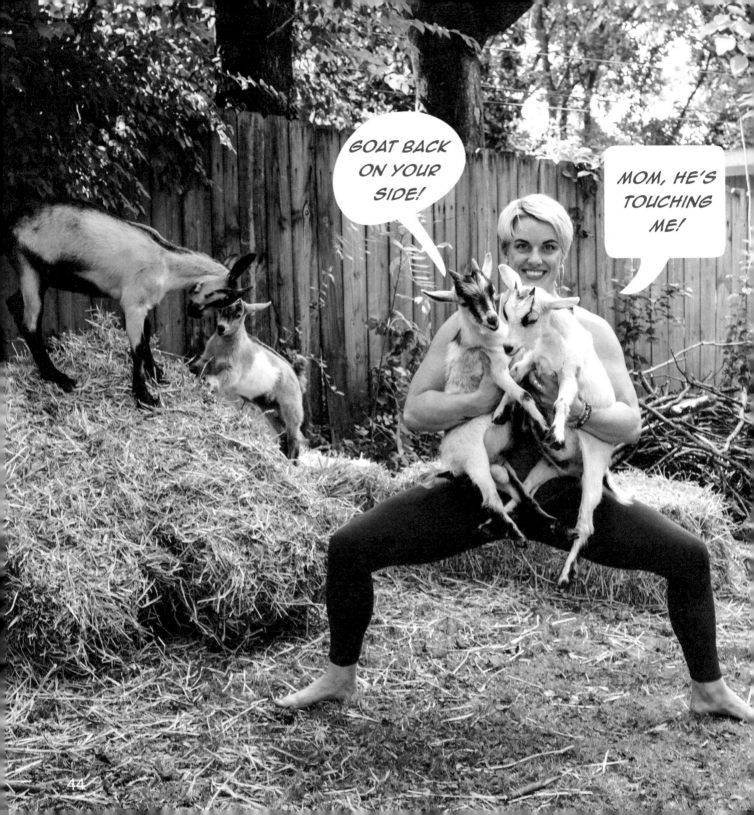

GOATTESS

(Goddess)

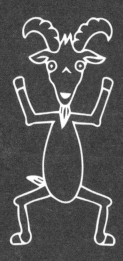

This variation of Goddess requires twin goats and one very strong yogi. Using core, leg, and arm strength, you'll need to remember to hold onto your goats—just not too tight!

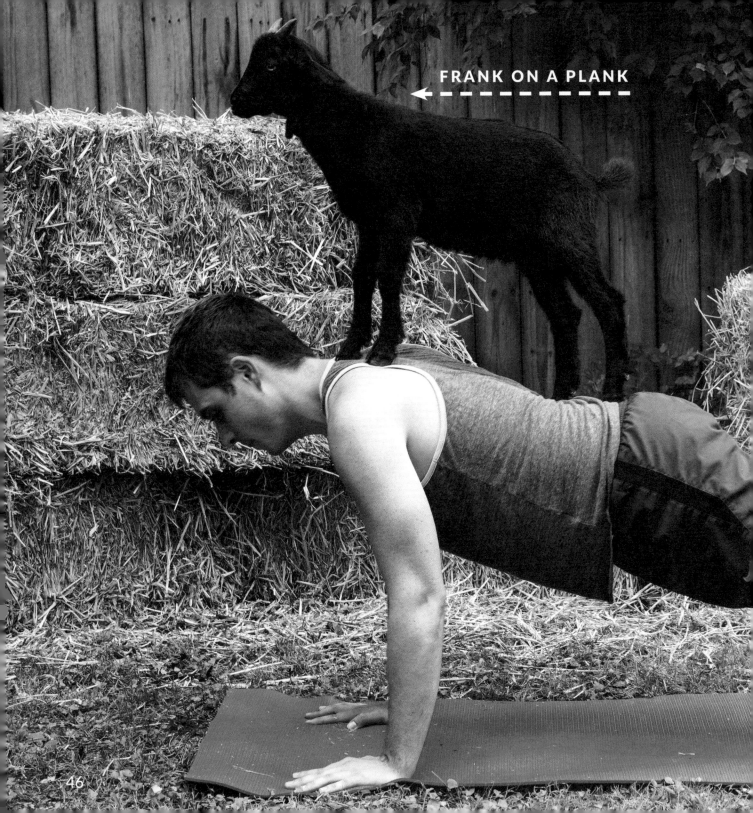

FRANK ON A PLANK

46

WALK THE GOAT PLANK
(Plank)

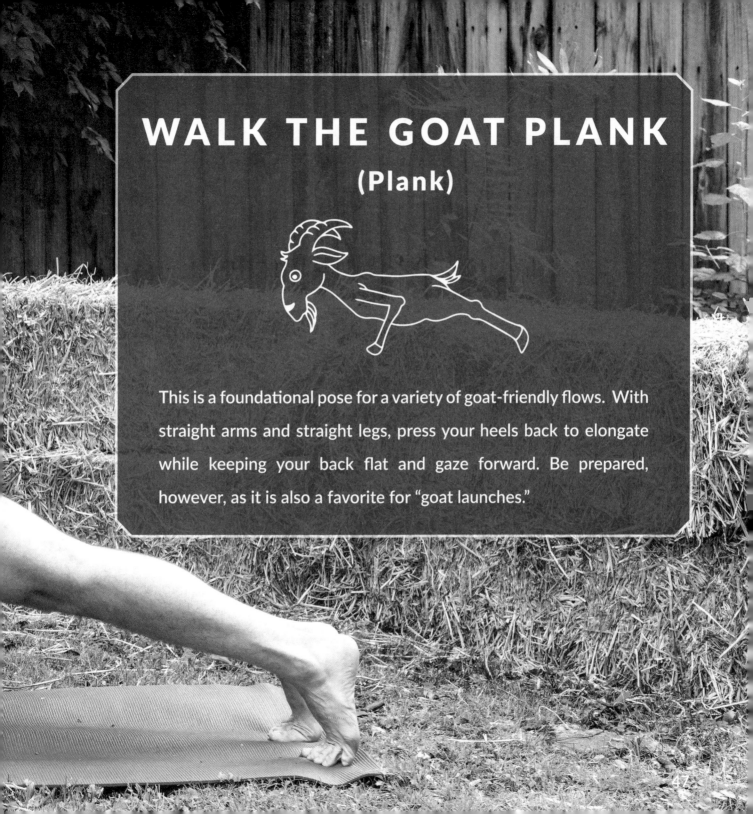

This is a foundational pose for a variety of goat-friendly flows. With straight arms and straight legs, press your heels back to elongate while keeping your back flat and gaze forward. Be prepared, however, as it is also a favorite for "goat launches."

ONE-LEGGED WALK THE GOAT PLANK

(One-Legged Plank)

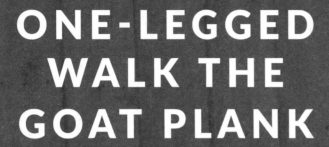

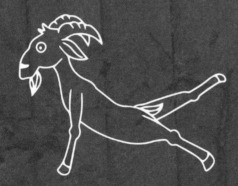

To jazz up your plank, you can alternate lifting your arms and legs and/or accessorizing your goat partners. Always check for goats before lowering into chaturanga.

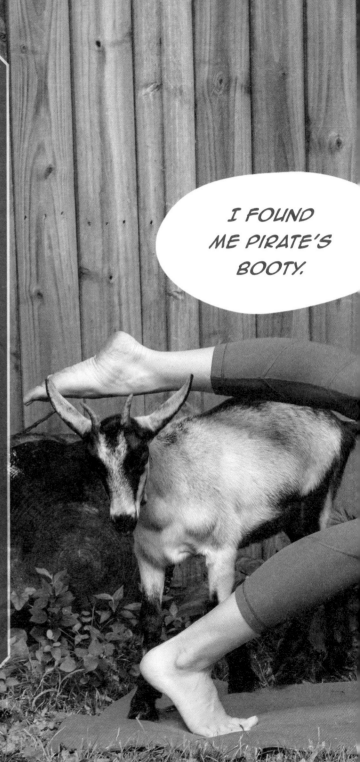

I FOUND ME PIRATE'S BOOTY.

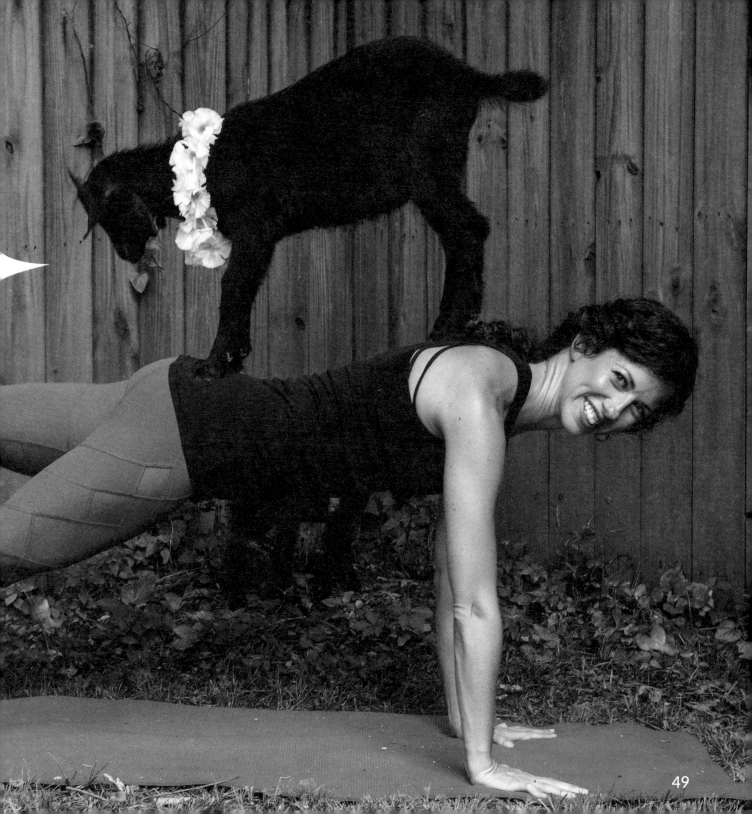

HORN TO KNEE POSE

(Standing Forehead to Knee)

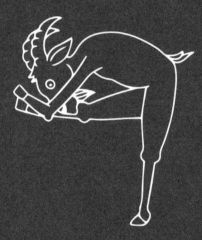

This challenging pose tests strength, balance, and flexibility and, once perfected, provides the perfect perch for a deep goat back massage. To release your goat, lower your lifted leg to meet your standing leg.

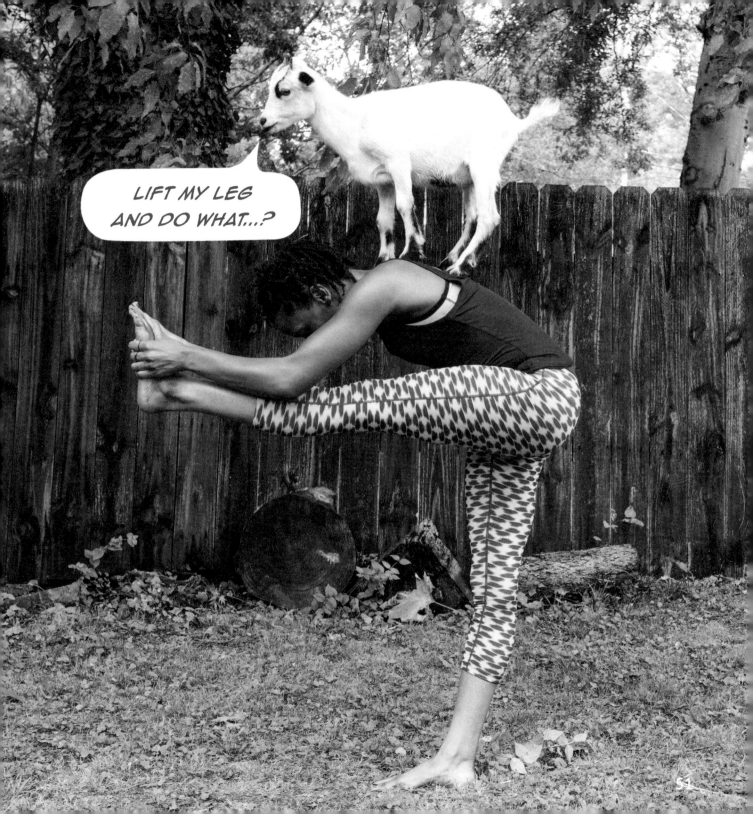

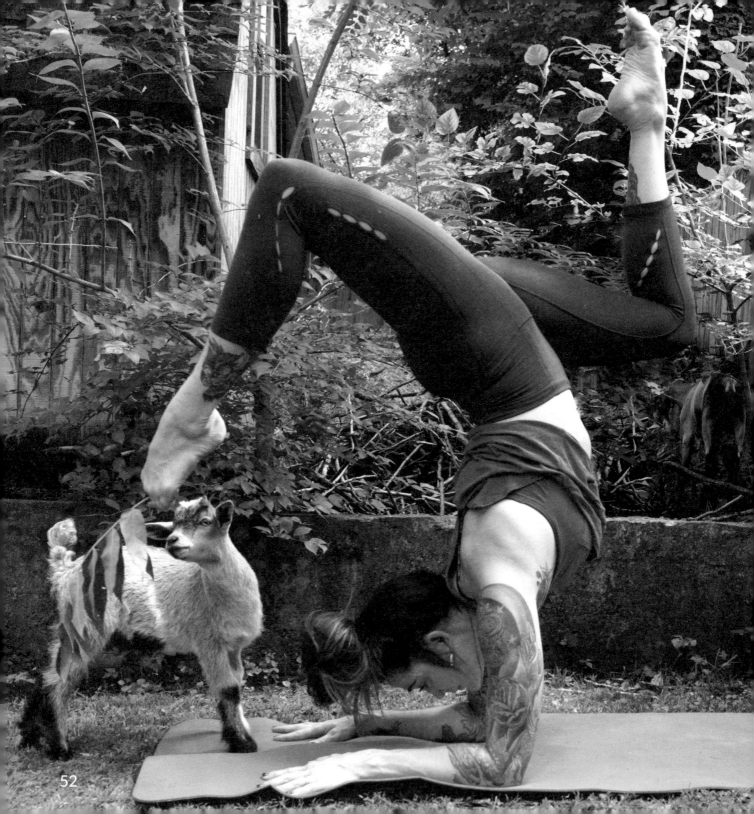

UPSIDE DOWN, GOATSIDE UP
(Inversion)

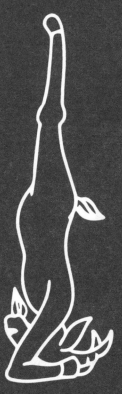

Inversions are some of the most beneficial goat yoga poses, but make sure that you can successfully invert before adding a goat! Inversion calms the mind, strengthens the whole body, and is an incredible photo op as this pose provides one of the highest perches for the most advanced cloven yogis.

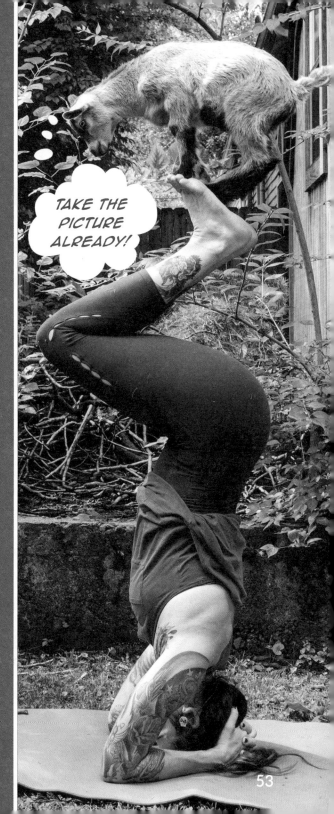

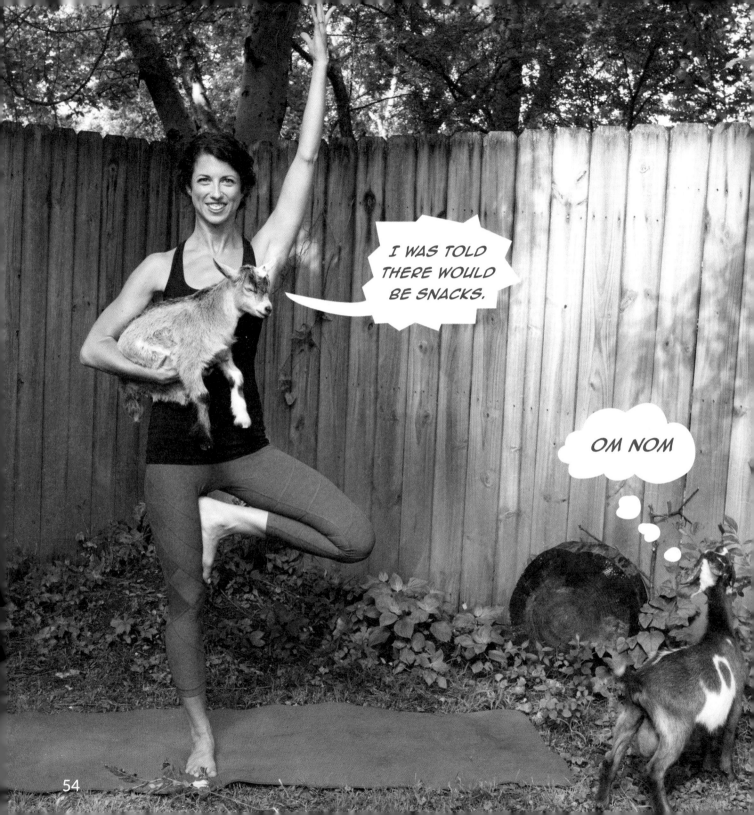

GOAT IN A TREE
(Tree)

Goats are expert climbers and are known to climb trees to forage for the best leaves. This tree is more about balance and is a great mid-practice pose to center yourself and your goat. With a strong standing leg, bend your other leg to set your foot against either your calf or thigh, but never your knee. Your arms can feel free to move as the mood, and goat, suits you.

WILD GOAT THANG

(Wild Thing)

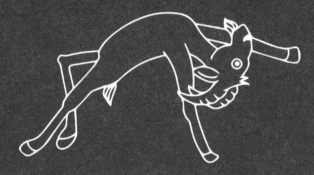

A fun, energizing and uplifting pose, this backbend out of Downward Facing Goat (page 24) provides another fun perch for feeding hungry goats. Make sure to keep your chest lifted to provide a stable and safe place for your goat to hang out— and remember to smile.

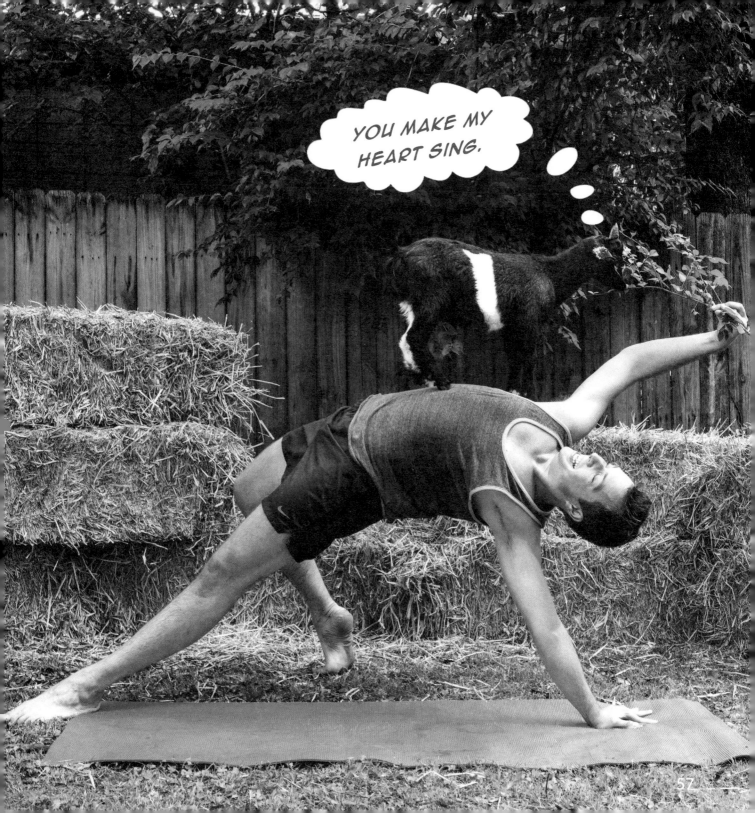

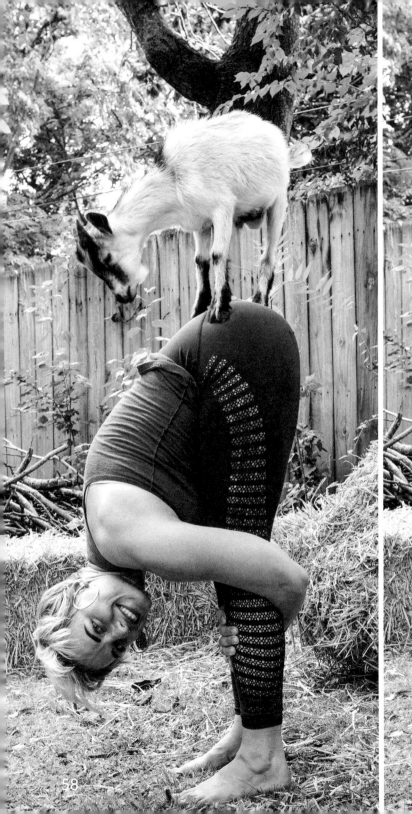
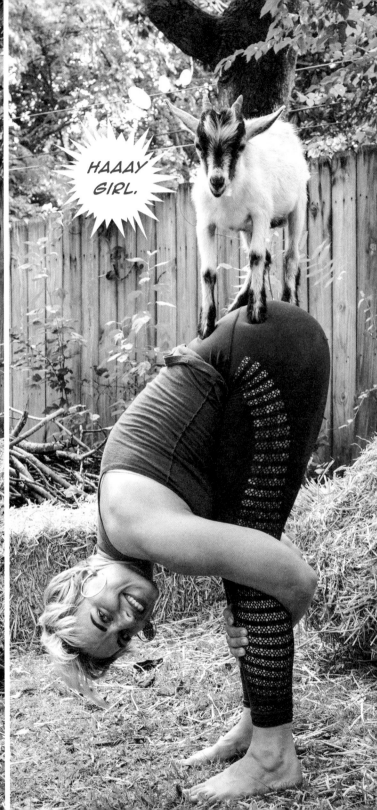

GOATDOLL

(Ragdoll)

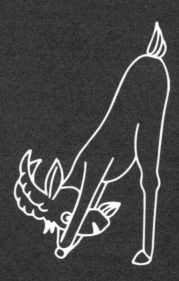

This classic forward fold is ideal for mountain goats and is a great way to relieve back tension. Feel free to let your arms hang or hug the back of your knees, and ham it up for the camera!

BOW PEEP

(Floor Bow)

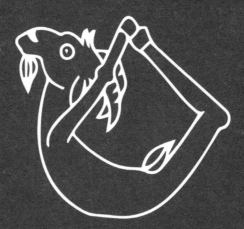

A great goat cradling pose. Lying on your stomach, reach back to grasp your ankles. Kick into your hands to lift your chest and knees off the ground. If you're lucky, you might grab a goat smooch!

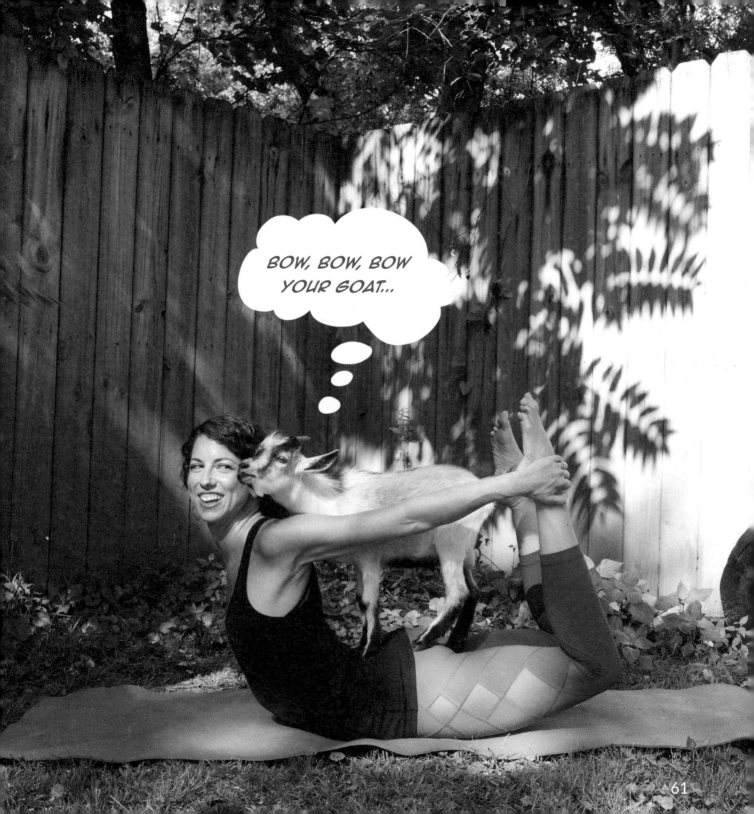

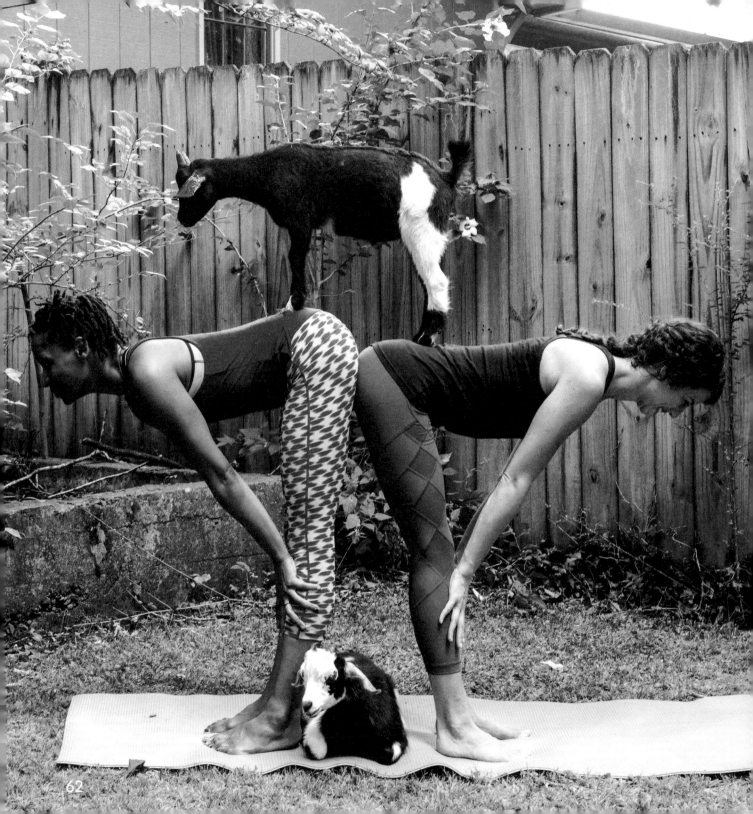

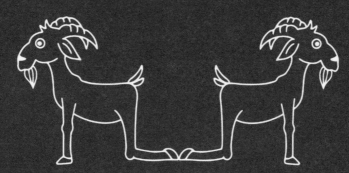

FLOWING WITH FRIENDS

Partner Poses and Acroyoga

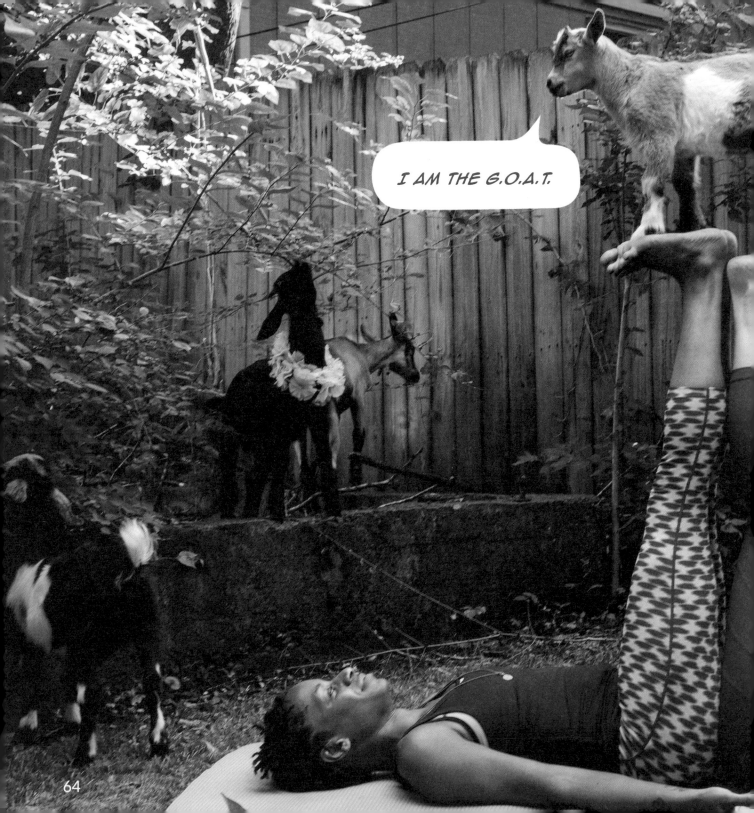

TROPHY GOAT

(Waterfall)

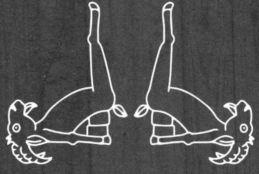

This restorative pose is great practiced alone against a wall or mirrored with a partner. It is a low-impact way to honor your MVP by hoisting him high.

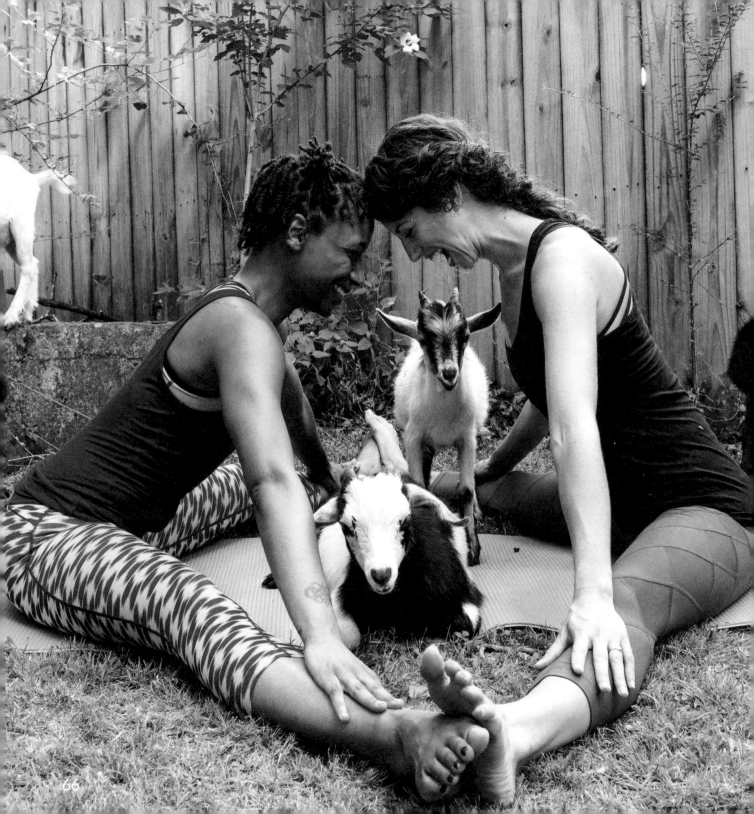

HEAD-BUTT
(Wide-Legged Forward Fold)

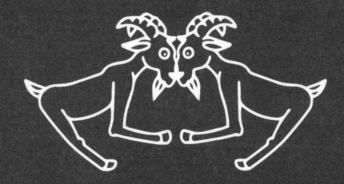

This partner variation plays off of a goat's favorite activity—head butting! Sitting mirrored with wide legs, bend forward to meet your partner and wait for the goats to follow suit!

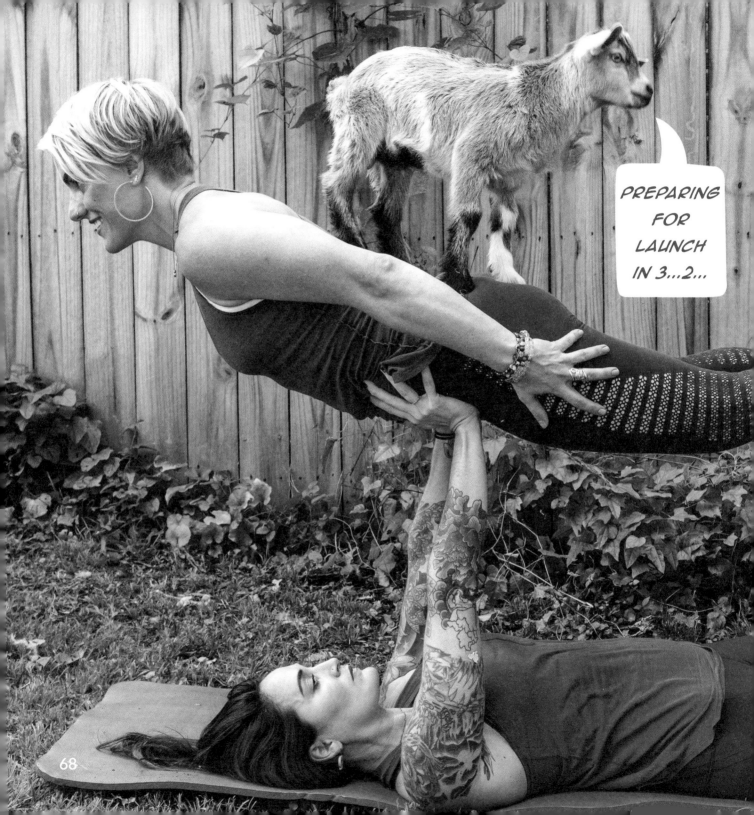

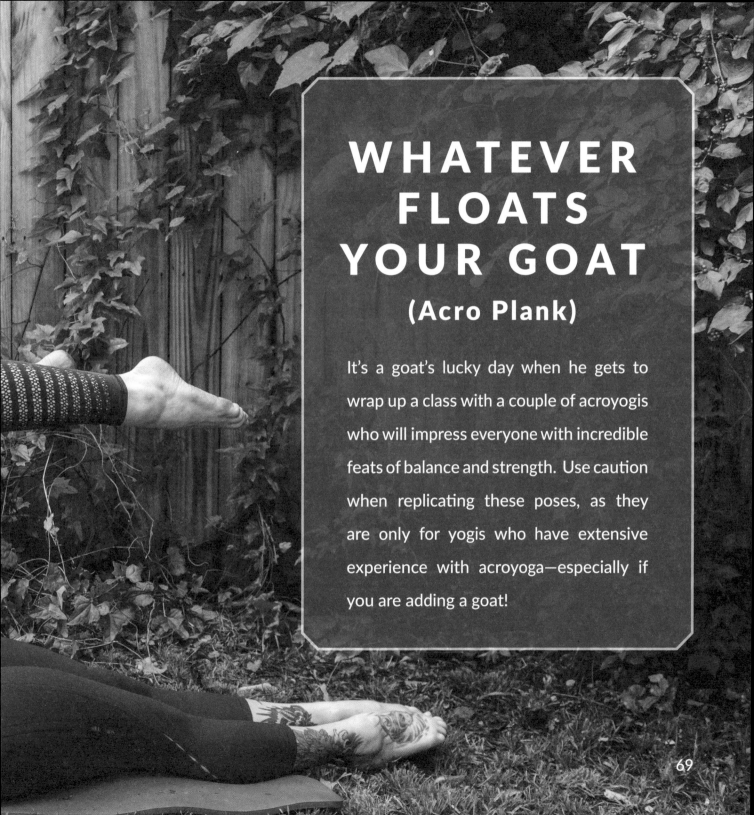

WHATEVER FLOATS YOUR GOAT

(Acro Plank)

It's a goat's lucky day when he gets to wrap up a class with a couple of acroyogis who will impress everyone with incredible feats of balance and strength. Use caution when replicating these poses, as they are only for yogis who have extensive experience with acroyoga—especially if you are adding a goat!

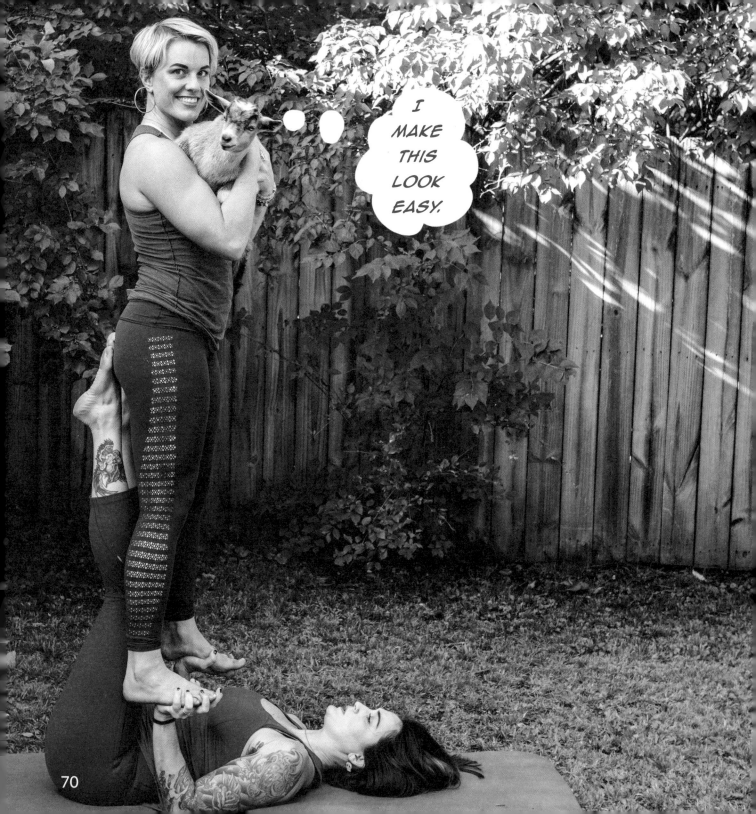

MOUNTAIN GOAT

(Tadasana Acro)

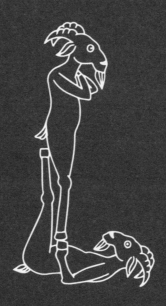

This is definitely a pose that looks easier than it is for both yogis. The base yogi must have unflinching core strength while the standing yogi must be balanced and calm (and it doesn't hurt to find a docile goat, either). So, keep calm and goat on!

SPIRIT ANIMAL
(Side Plank Acro)

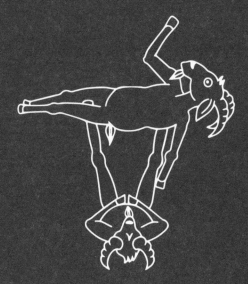

Goat yogis must always remember that their greatest assets are the four-legged friends that make this wonderful practice possible. We may not understand why goats and yoga make such a perfect pairing, but we are surely thankful for their willing participation.

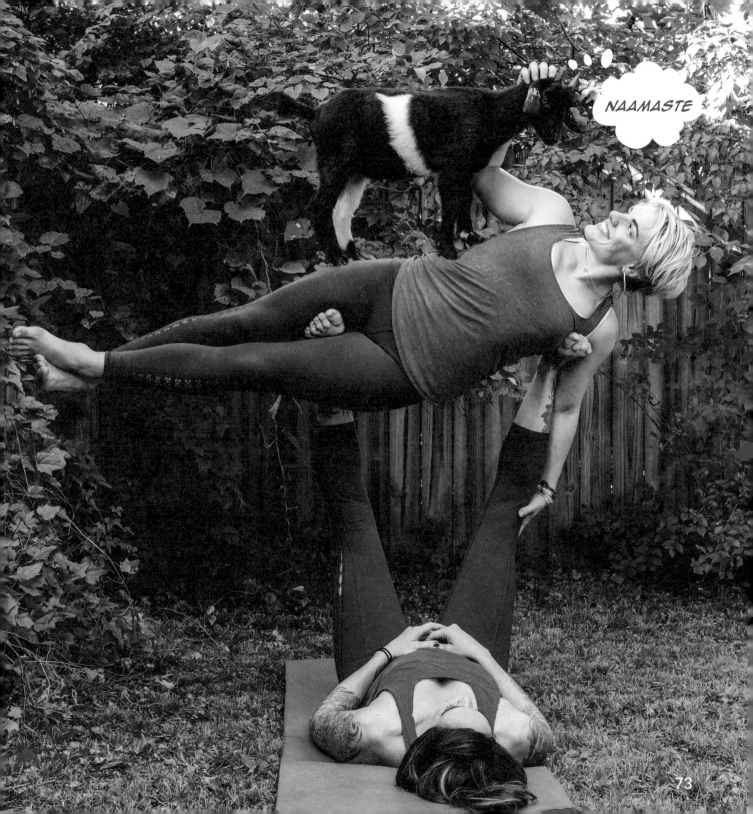

73

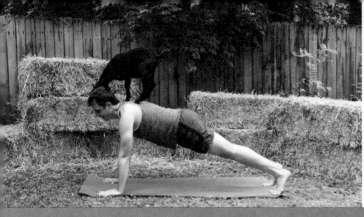
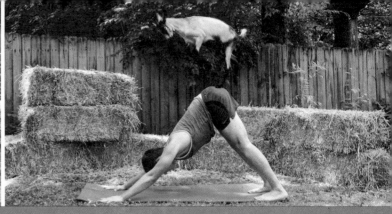

WELCOME TO THE

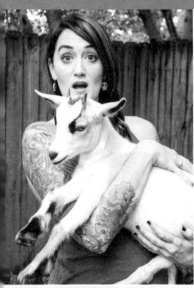
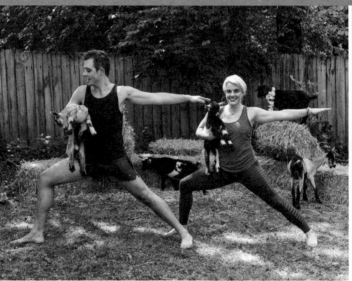
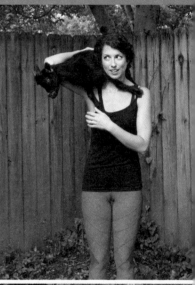

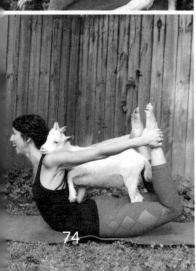

74

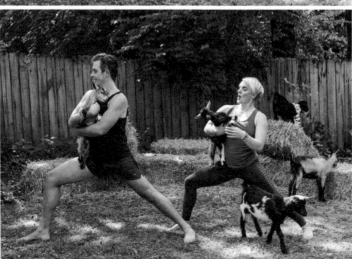
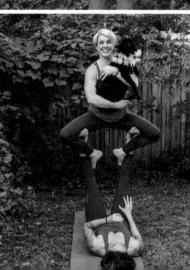

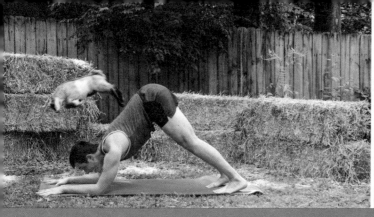
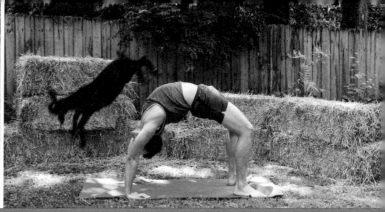

GOAT RODEO!

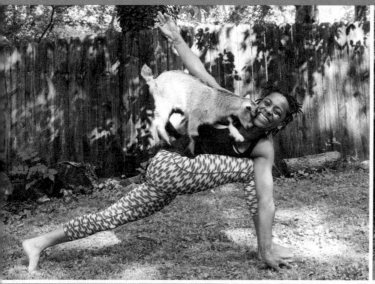
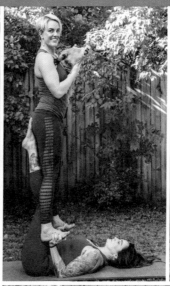
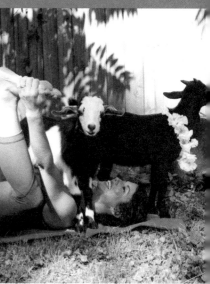
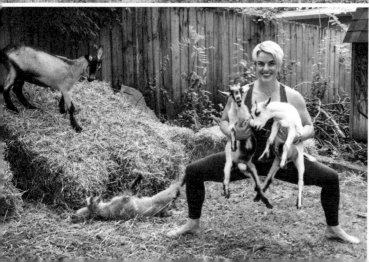
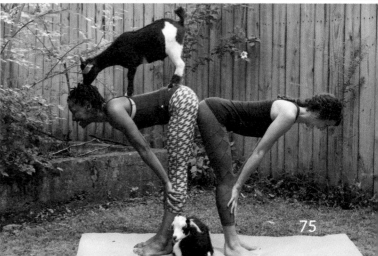

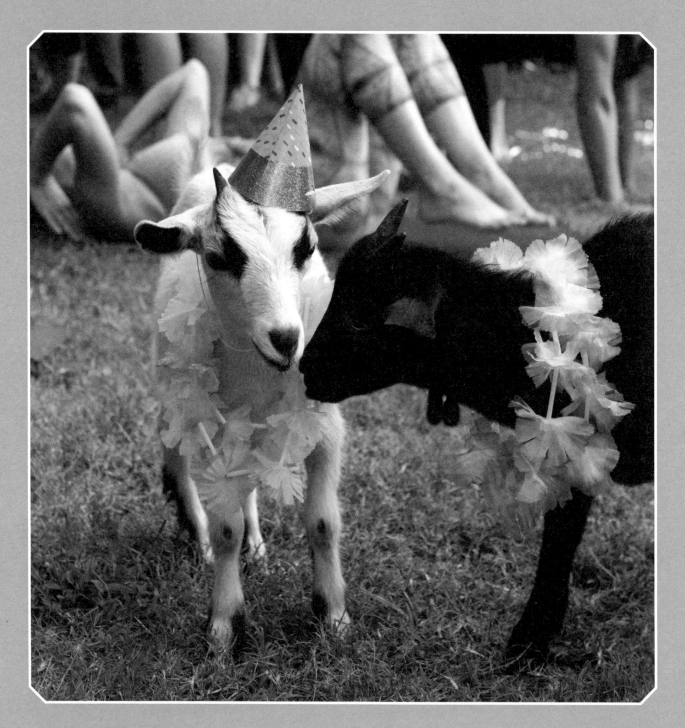

GOAT YOGA | YOGA ALL DAY, PARTY ALL NIGHT!

YOGA ALL DAY, PARTY ALL NIGHT!

How to Throw an Amazing Goat Yoga Party

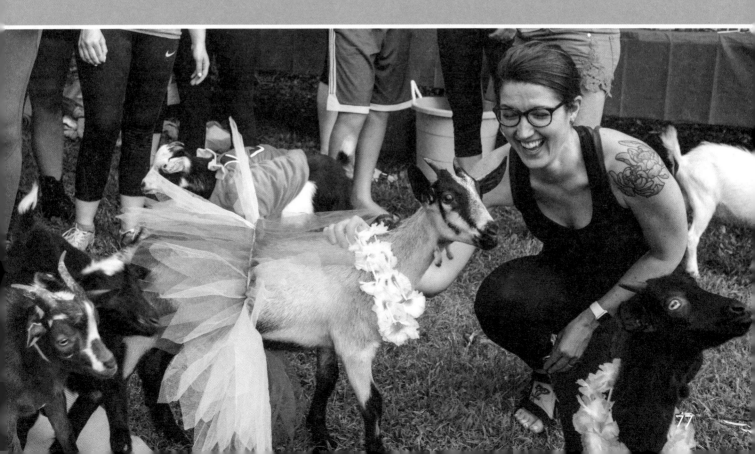

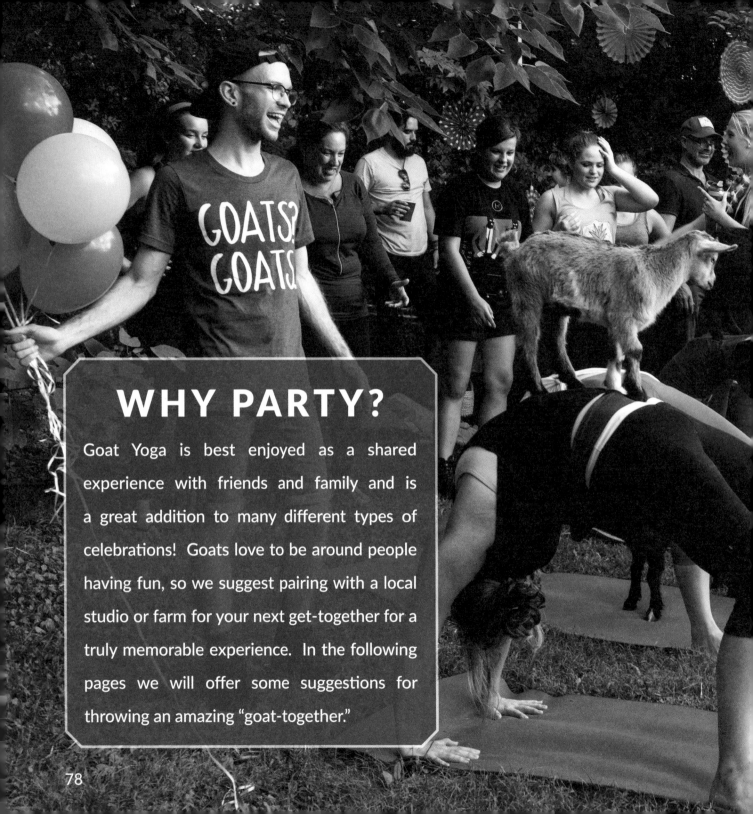

WHY PARTY?

Goat Yoga is best enjoyed as a shared experience with friends and family and is a great addition to many different types of celebrations! Goats love to be around people having fun, so we suggest pairing with a local studio or farm for your next get-together for a truly memorable experience. In the following pages we will offer some suggestions for throwing an amazing "goat-together."

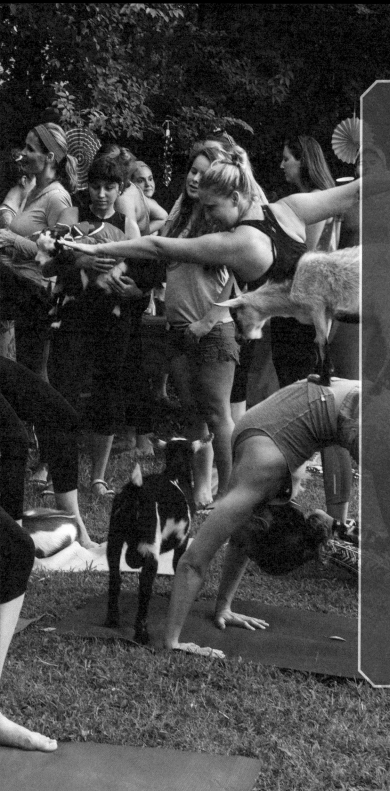

WHAT KIND OF CELEBRATIONS?

- Birthdays
- Engagement Parties
- Employee Parties
- Bachelorette/Bachelor Parties
- Open Houses
- Album/Book Release Parties
- Housewarmings
- Gender Reveal Parties
- Wine Tastings
- Studio Openings
- Charity Events
- Divorce Parties
- TGIF

ETIQUETTE

Just because you are partying with goats doesn't mean that you need to act like you were raised in a barn. Goat Yoga is a very unique experience that can be added to many different occasions, but there are a few things that you should remember...

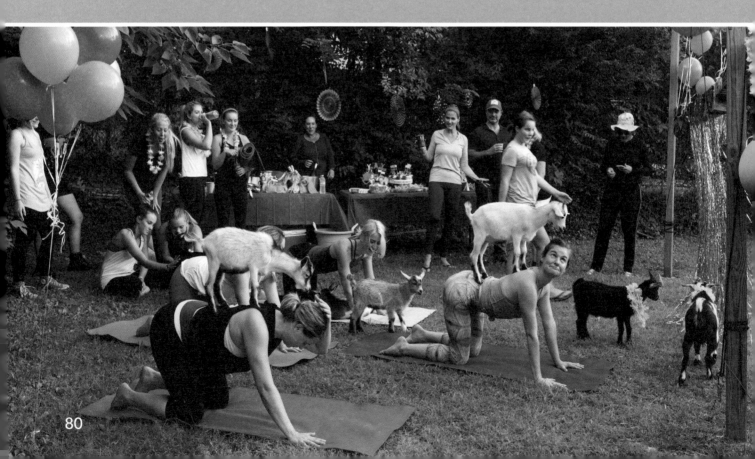

MIND YOUR P'S AND GOATS

- Don't bring your dog without asking first.
- Wear comfortable clothing, but remember that you'll be photographed—A LOT.
- Keep an eye on your party accessories—goats like to dress up, but they also try to eat almost anything.
- Don't forget to offer a lot of praise for the goats—if they're happy, you're happy.
- Leave your reservations at home—get on the mat and take a photo with that goat!
- Please imbibe around the goats, but not with them.
- If you see something, say something—maybe she doesn't know that she is about to step in a pile of...
- Take photos for your neighbors and share them after class. It's a great conversation starter and a wonderful way to make new friends whose interests are as wacky as yours!

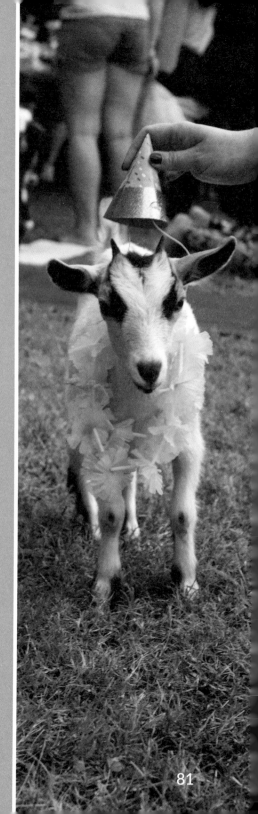

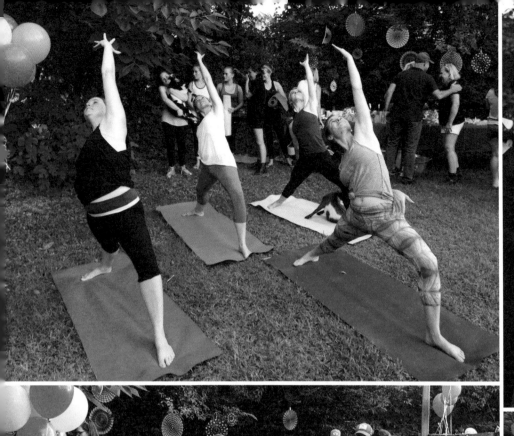

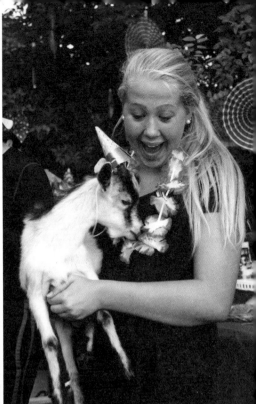

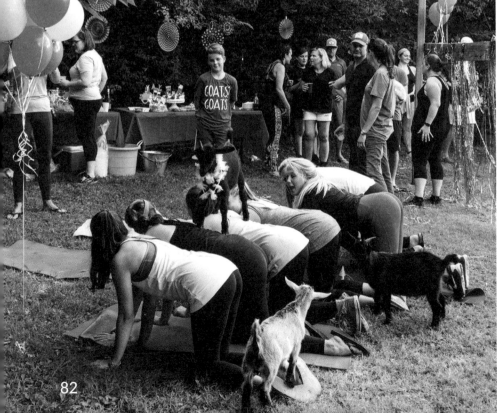

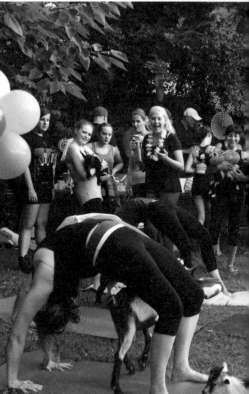

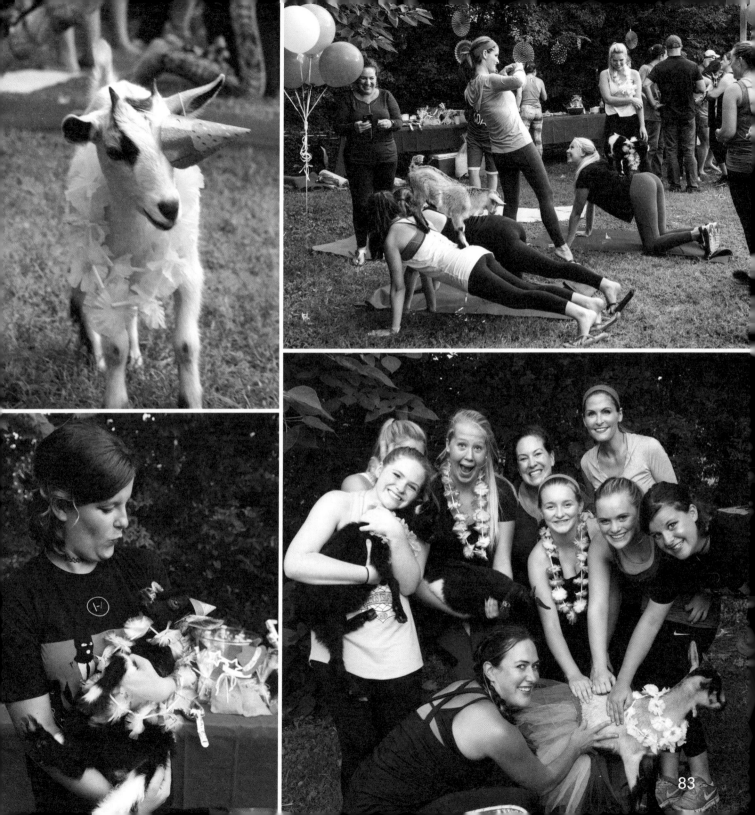

WHAT TO SERVE

Depending on the setting and occasion, a goat yoga party can be accompanied by a variety of treats! We suggest finding as many goat-friendly snacks as possible that can be shared by all attendees (cloven or otherwise). A vegetable platter and fresh apples will be a hit for the goats, while goat-adorned cupcakes and themed beverages will delight the bipedal attendees.

Party favor suggestions: wet wipes, photo booth props, raisins and dried fruit, bubbles.

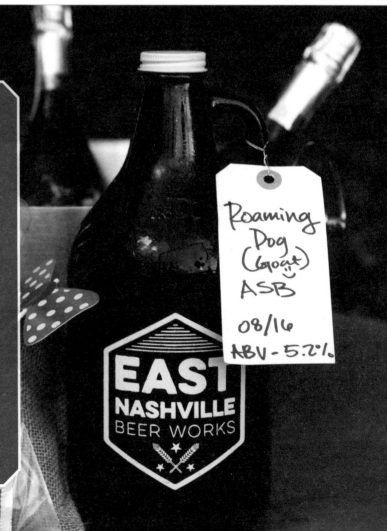

Goatmeal Cookies
By Chef Matt Clement

Ingredients:
- 1 ½ sticks Unsalted Butter, fluid and warm
- 1 tablespoon Vanilla Extract
- 1 Egg, cold
- ¾ cup, gently packed Brown Sugar
- 1 cup Granulated White Sugar
- 2 teaspoons Kosher Salt
- 1 teaspoon Ground Cinnamon
- 1/2 teaspoon Baking Soda
- 2 cups Old-Fashioned Rolled Oats—not quick-cooking or instant
- 1 ¼ cups All-Purpose Flour
- 1 ¼ cups Dried Cranberries or Cherries

Method:

1.) Adjust oven rack to middle position, preheat to 350°F, and line pans with parchment.

2.) Combine butter, vanilla, egg, brown sugar, white sugar, kosher salt, cinnamon, and baking soda in a medium bowl. Stir until no lumps remain, then fold in rolled oats, followed by the flour and dried cranberries or cherries. Divide into 30 one-ounce portions with a roughly 2-tablespoon scoop and arrange on prepared sheet pans. Ideally, the dough will now be refrigerated overnight, or 8 hours. At the very least, let the dough stand at room temperature for at least 25 minutes, no more than 75.

3.) Bake until pale gold around the edges, but still puffed and steamy in the center, about 15 minutes. Cool directly on sheet pans until firm, about 10 minutes. Enjoy warm, or store in airtight container up to 3 days at room temperature.

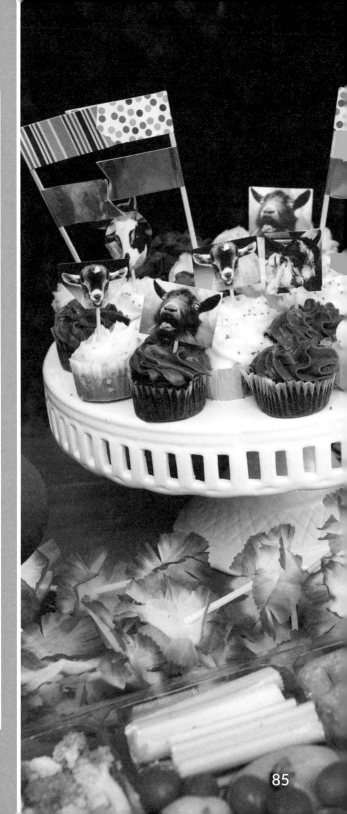

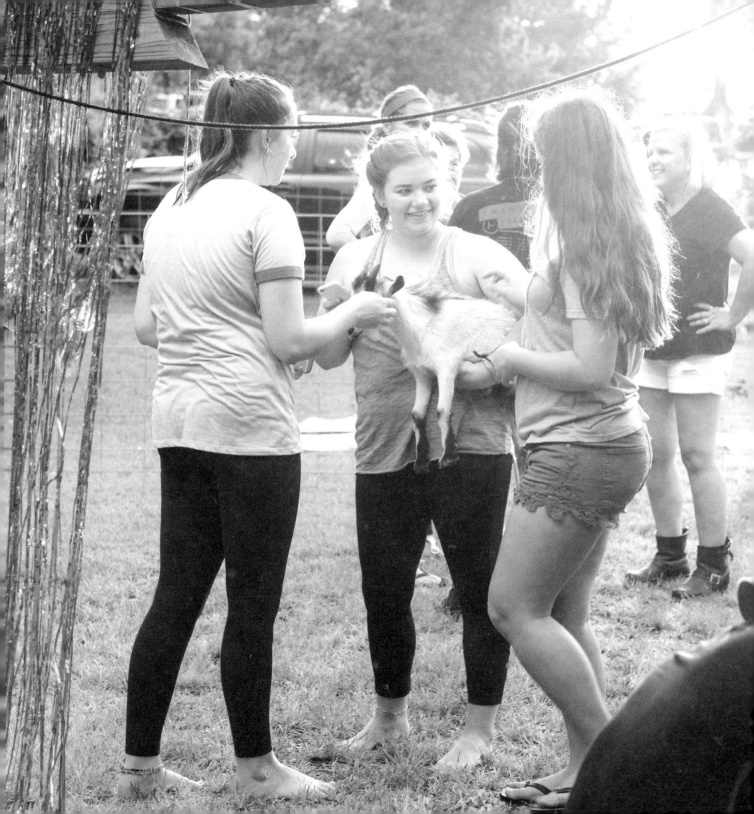

ACKNOWLEDGEMENTS

Shenanigoats would like to thank our families, our seemingly tireless team (Shane and Mush, Kesley, Elizabeth, Kyle, Sheila, Stephen, Ari, Abbey, Karin, and Liz)—we are so aware that we need each of you to make this all happen and we are forever thankful for you. Stephanie, for turning a plain garage into the perfect goat studio —you created the most amazing space. Dirt Floor Productions—we so appreciate your patience with us and your ability to just get it done. To our instructors (Lori, Brianne, Andi, Raquel, Kelly, Meredith, Sara Jane, Janaye, Gillian, and Jenna) who give it their all in each class amid the distraction of laughter, selfies, and poop. Lin— we love you so much and still owe you red hots—about 100 cases worth. Our first cheerleaders, Bethany, Jessica, and Ben. We want to thank every goat farmer out there whose work never ends, to the families and farmers that trusted us to raise their kids, to Kate and Mike for letting us provide our goats in their educational process. Thank you to Fred and Sarah for your unique talents—truly unexpected friends. Thank you to all of those who have provided us space and support. Thank you Lindy and Bo, Paula and Cindy, Nashville Guru, Do615, and Casie and Kristen at NewsChannel 5 for helping us move faster down this path and for having faith in us and our kids. Thank you Leslie, Rob, and Doug...your insane talent and drive is a true example to us. Most importantly, we want to thank each other—our winding road has led us to this point and we wouldn't change a thing. We are beyond grateful for this journey and continue to be humbled with each leap.

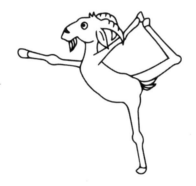

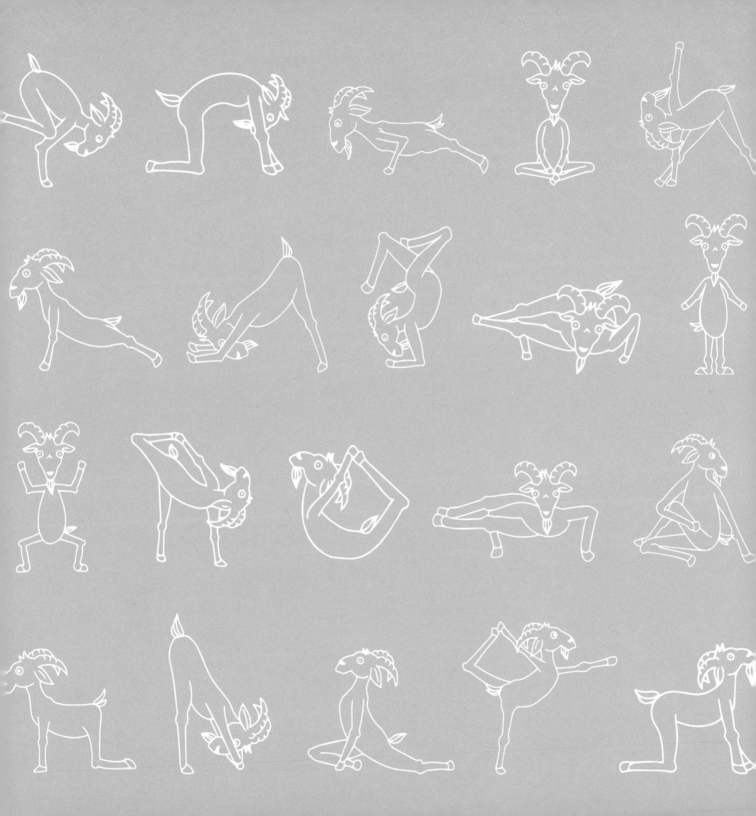